ALCHEMY AND METALLIC MEDICINES IN AYURVEDA

By the Same Author Published by **CONCEPT**

TODARANANDA-AYURVEDA SAUKHYAM SERIES

No. 1 Materia Medica of Ayurveda

No. 2 Basic Principles of Ayurveda

No. 3 Diagnosis and Treatment of Diseases in Ayurveda (Part One)

No. 4 Diagnosis and Treatment of Diseases in Ayurveda (Part Two)

No. 5 Diagnosis and Treatment of Diseases in Ayurveda (Part Three)

No. 6 Diagnosis and Treatment of Diseases in Ayurveda (Part Four)

No. 7 Diagnosis and Treatment of Diseases in Ayurved (Part Five)

No. 8 Five Specialist Therapies of Ayurveda *(Pancha-Karma)*

No. 9 Iatro-Chemistry of Ayurveda *(Rasa Sastra)*

A Handbook of Ayurveda (The Handbook has been published in *Italian* and *Japanese* edition)

Message Therapy in Ayurveda (*Pancha-Karma Therapy of Ayurveda Series* No. 1)

About the Author

Vaidya Bhagwan Dash has had an outstandingly brilliant academic career. He holds a Master's degree and a doctorate from Delhi University in addition to postgraduate qualifications in Ayurveda.

A Sanskrit scholar, he handles the English language with equal felicity. A significant advantage to his propensity for research in Ayurveda is Dr. Dash's proficiency in Tibetan, German, French and Mongolian. In the course of nearly twenty-five years dedicated to research in and the practice of Ayurveda, Dr. Dash has attended several important conferences and seminars both in India and abroad. He has also contributed innumerable articles to reputed national and international journals in indology, medicine and science.

The author of many important publications covering several aspects of Ayurveda and Tibetan medicine, he has to his credit three volumes of an English translation of *Caraka Saṃhitā*, an ancient Ayurveda classic. He was recently on a short-term assignment as WHO Consultant in Traditional Medicine to the Government of Bhutan.

He was working as Deputy Adviser (Ayurveda) to the Government of India in the Ministry of Health and Family Welfare till 31 May 1981, when he took voluntary retirement with a view to enable him to devote more time for academic and research work.

ALCHEMY
AND
METALLIC MEDICINES
IN
AYURVEDA

by

VAIDYA BHAGWAN DASH

D.A.M.S., H.P.A., M.A., Ph.D.

CONCEPT PUBLISHING COMPANY, NEW DELHI-110059

ISBN 81-7022-077-7

First Published 1986
Reprinted 1996, 2003

Published and Printed by
Ashok Kumar Mittal
Concept Publishing Company
A/15-16, Commercial Block, Mohan Garden
NEW DELHI-110059 (India)

Phones : 25351460, 25351794
Fax : 091-11-25357103
Email : publishing@conceptpub.com

CONTENTS

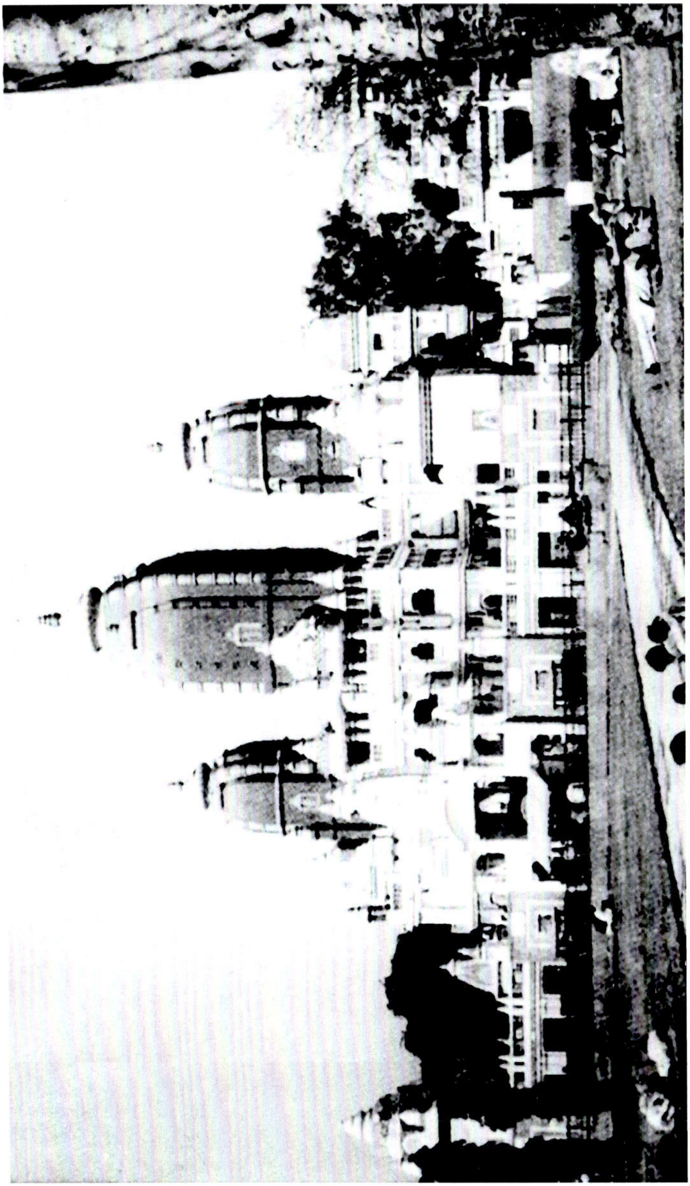

1 Lakshmi Narayana Temple (popularly known as Birla Temple) in New Delhi in which compound alchemical experiments on mercury were carried out.

(Facing Page 24-25)

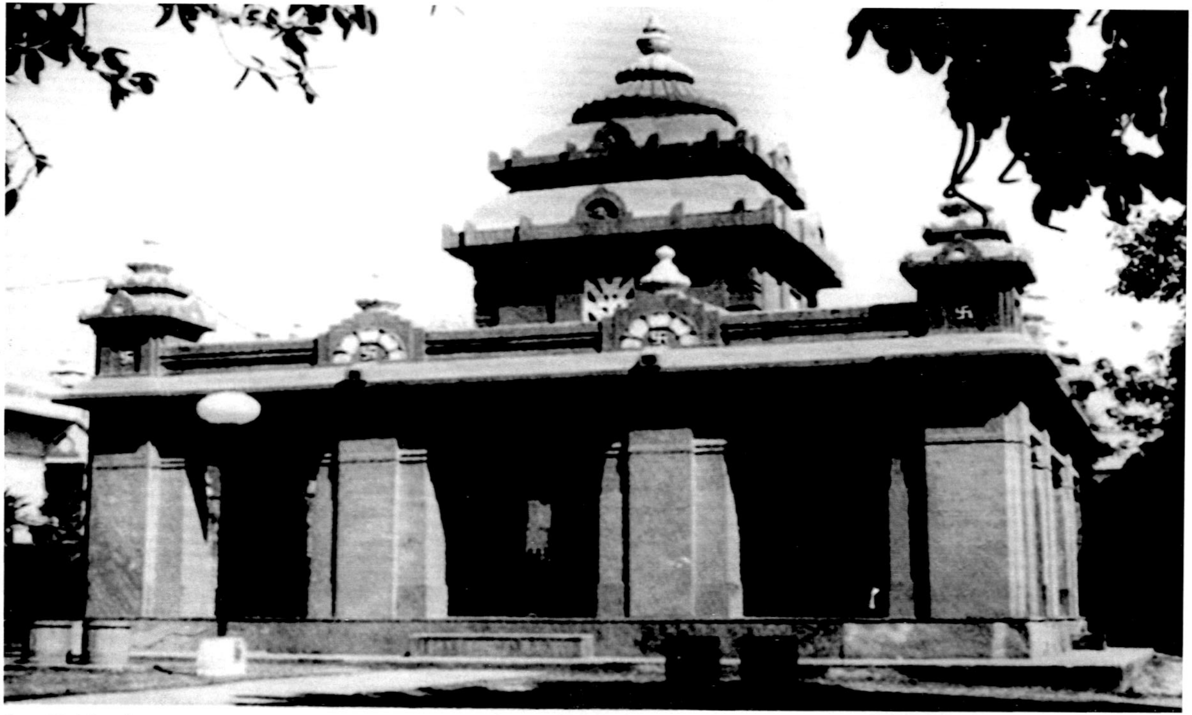

2 Yajña-śala of Birla Temple in the pillars of which details of alchemical processes are engraved.

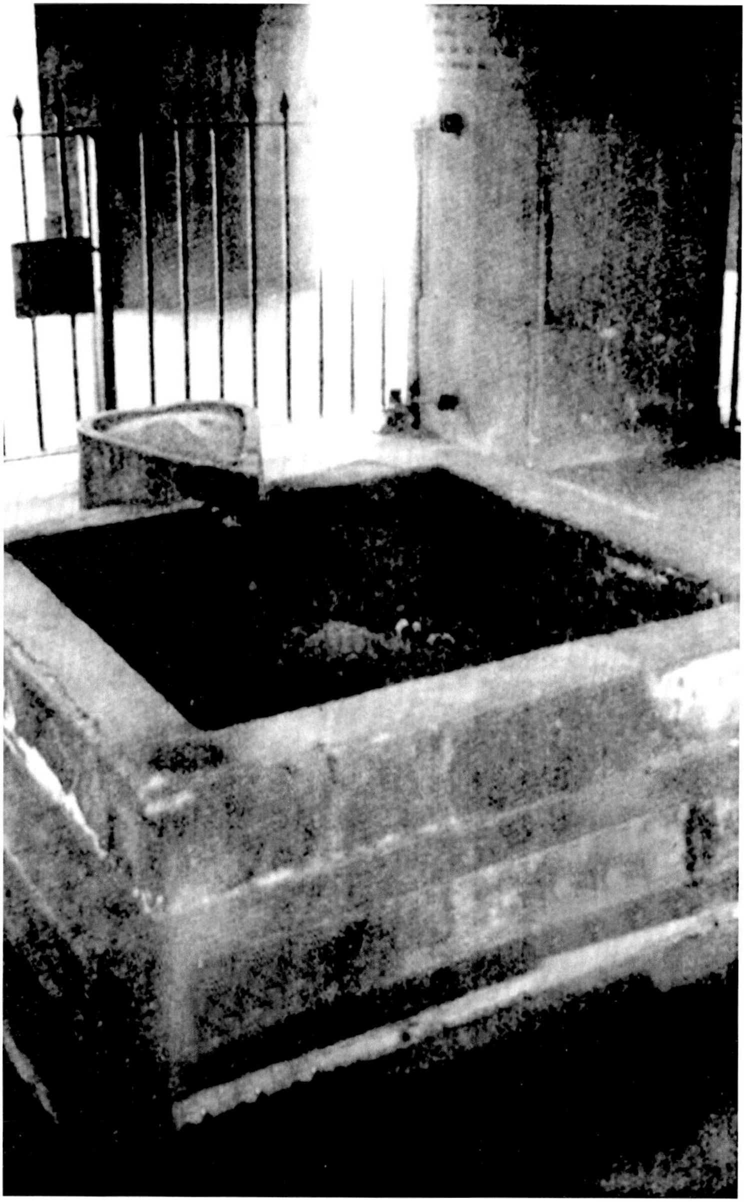

3 Yajña-Kuṇḍa with a part of the pillar having inscriptions.

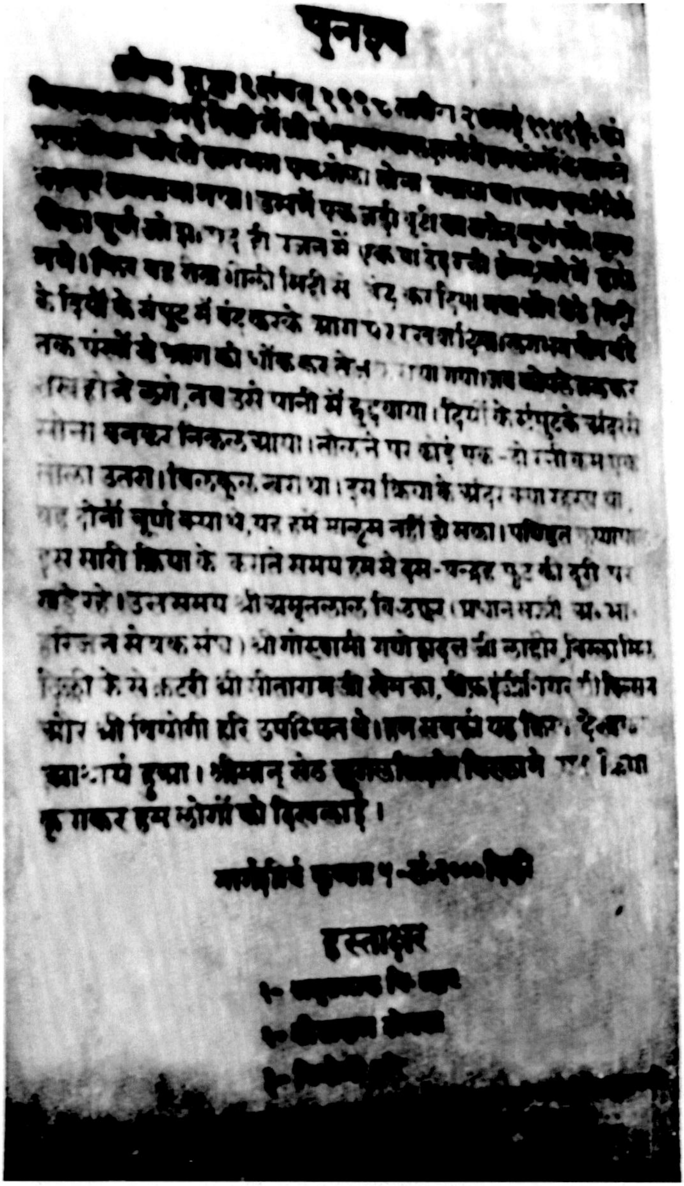

4 **One of the inscriptions giving details of the alchemical process in Hindi.**

LIST OF PLATES AND FIGURES

Plates

Figures

INDO-ROMANIC EQUIVALENTS OF DEVANĀGARĪ

Devanāgarī	Indo-Romanic	Devanāgarī	Indo-Romanic
अ	— a	ठ	— ṭha
आ	— ā	ड	— da
इ	— i	ढ	— ḍha
ई	— ī	ण	— ṇa
उ	— u	त	— ta
ऊ	— ū	थ	— tha
ऋ	— ṛ	द	— da
ए	— e	ध	— dha
ऐ	— ai	न	— na
	— ṃ	प	— pa
:	— ḥ	फ	— pha
क	— ka	ब	— ba
ख	— kha	भ	— bha
ग	— ga	म	— ma
घ	— gha	य	— ya
ङ	— ṅa	र	— ra
च	— ca	ल	— la
छ	— cha	व	— va
ज	— ja	श	— śa
झ	— jha	ष	— ṣa
ञ	— ña	स	— sa
ट	— ṭa	ह	— ha

PREFACE

Man's eternal endeavour has been to discover new things specially in the unexplored fields. It is this human effort which has culminated in the discovery of Alchemical methods and methods for utilisation of metals as well as minerals for therapeutic purposes. The term 'Alchemy' has been interpreted variously by different people. Some modern scientists have discredited this term to the extent of suggesting that it is a myth which man has never succeeded to achieve but for which he has always attempted. Alchemy was in practice in different European countries also. Some scholars claim success and others consider them to be false and quackery. It basically revolves round the preparation of noble metals like gold and silver from out of base metals like mercury and copper. Whatever may be the opinion in European countries, in India, it is not considered as a myth.

As early as 6th Century B.C. Cāṇakaya, an authority on statecraft had described in his monumental work *Arthaśāstra,* a type of gold which was prepared by *vedha* (transmutation) of base metals with processed mercury, and he had termed this type of gold as *rasa vedha svarṇa.* It is very clear from this description that alchemy was in practice, rather successful practice, in India even before 6th Century B.C. In subsequent works on *rasa śāstra* (Iatro-Chemistry) different methods have been described for processing mercury with a view to making it capable of transmuting base metals into gold and silver. These descriptions are so cryptic that for ordinary scholars, it becomes difficult of comprehension. Different stages of the processing are intentionally kept secret and often some descriptions are made which give different meanings. This is done largely because the propounders and patrons of these methods did not want the knowledge to go to unscruplous persons who may amass wealth by the practice of this technique to indulge themselves in anti-social activities.

Alchemy, according to Indian tradition, is not an end in itself. It is only a means. The actual intention of processing mercury is to administer it for the preservation and promotion of positive rites unhindered for a sufficiently long period to achieve *jīvan mukti* i.e. salvation from the bondage of the world while remaining alive. To ascertain the suitability of mercury for administration to an individual, it is tested over raw (unprocessed) mercury and other base metals. If it is capable of transmutation of ordinary mercury into gold then it is considered to be suitable for administration to the individual. This method is still in practice secretly by saints who are adept in this science. In 1949, a saint by name Pt. Kṛṣṇa Lāla Śarmā and the fifth chapter of this work is based on these discussions held and notes taken by the author.

In present day medical practice, Ayurvedic physicians profusely use metals, minerals, gems, jewels and animal as well as vegetable products which in raw form are well known to produce toxicity. Intellectuals of India and scientists of abroad naturally question the wisdom of using such toxic drugs for therapeutic purposes. This is largely because of their ignorance about the rationality of the methods of processing of these poisonous drugs before they are actually used in medicines.

In English and in nontechnical language, books on this topic are rare. Some earlier attempts in this connection have unfortunately made this confusion worst confounded because of mistranslation of certain technical terms. Translation of these technical terms into English is, no doubt, a difficult task. In Ayurveda, these terms carry subtle meanings for which equivalents are not available in English. These terms, therefore, need explanation and not mere translation.

As Physics and Chemistry explain the rationality of different drugs used in modern medicines, similarly the appropriateness of the processing followed by Ayurvedic physicians to make metals, etc. free from toxicity and to potentise them to achieve therapeutic excellence is explained by saints in Indian philosophical works.

In the introduction to the work, the utility of metals and minerals for prevention as well as cure of the diseases and preservation as well as promotion of positive health has been explained.

The First chapter deals with the historical background explaining the origin of *Rasa śāstra* and its subsequent development during the Buddhistic and medieval periods. Some important extant texts along with their authors are chronologically described.

The Second chapter explains the physico-chemical and philosophical concepts basic to the *rasa śāstra*. This explains the rationality of various processes like *śodhana* and *māraṇa* by which these metals and minerals are made non-toxic, absorbable, assimilable and therapeutically effective. The concept of *jīvan mukti* (salvation while remaining alive) and its significance are explained on the basis of philosophical concepts of Saivaites (one of the sects of the Hindus).

The Third chapter deals with the implications of the term *rasa* and the procedure to be adopted for the selection of site for the pharmaceutical laboratory, its construction, equipments as well as assistants.

Fourth chapter deals with mercury, its *doṣas* or defects because of which it produces toxicity in unprocessed form, and details of its processing. For the treatment of ordinary diseases, only eight *saṃskāras* (stages of processing) are considered to be enough. But to make it more potent for curing obstinate and otherwise incurable diseases and to make it more effective for the purpose of rejuvenation *(rasāyana)* which results in longevity leading to salvation while alive *(jīvan mukti)*, mercury should be subjected to eighteen stages which taken together are called *aṣṭādaśa saṃskāras*. *Deha-siddhi* (perfection of the body and mind of the individual) is the primary aim of using processed mercury. Before it is administered to a person the processed mercury is to be tested on metals. If this mercury could cause transmutation of base metals, like ordinary mercury into noble metals like gold and silver, only then it is considered suitable for *deha-siddhi*. Examining the processed mercury by the transmutation of base metals into noble metals is called *lauha-siddhi* (perfection in achieving transmutation of metals). As has been suggested before, this chapter, namely fourth is written on the basis of notes collected from one of the disciples of the saint Pt. Kṛṣṇa Lāla Śarmā. However, it will be seen from the descriptions in these two chapters that most of them are taken from extant texts on *Rasa śāstra* with, of course, certain modifications.

In the day-to-day practice, Ayurvedic physicians use several mercurial preparations. A few important recipes are described in the Fifth chapter. Normally, mercury is processed according to the eight stages *(aṣṭa saṃskāras)* before preparing the recipe. Some physicians and drug manufacturers, however, use simpler methods for processing by which mercury, no doubt, becomes free from toxicity but this type of mercury is not very effective when used in recipes. In addition to the recipes described in this chapter, several thousands of other mercurial compounds are used in ayurvedic practice. Generally, purified mercury and purified sulphur along with other metals, minerals and vegetable as well as animal products are added to these recipes.

Details of such recipes are not furnished in the present work. Any standard text on *Rasa śāstra* or *Bhaiṣajya kalpanā* will, however, provide information in this regard to inquisitive readers.

The Sixth chapter deals with other commonly used metals and minerals. Their synonyms, adverse effects when used in unprocessed form, *śodhana, māraṇa,* properties, therapeutic indications, dose and *anupāna* or vehicle are described. The primary aim of this book is to present before scholars an outline of methods followed by ancient Indian saints for processing mercury and other metals as well as minerals to make them suitable for the prevention and cure of diseases and for the preservation and promotion of positive health. Details are, therefore, avoided. Those interested in acquiring detailed knowledge on this topic can refer to extant texts on the subject. In the Seventh chapter, only the choisest methods of processing metals and minerals are described. In addition, ayurvedic physicians adopt several other methods. Some methods, they claim to be equal, if not better.

Like metals and minerals, gems and jewels are also used for the treatment of obstinate and otherwise incurable diseases. Most of these gems and jewels are, no doubt, minerals. But because of their specific characteristics, these are described separately in the Seventh chapter. The gems and jewels are, in addition, used astrologically to propitiate planatory bodies. A passing reference to this has been made in this chapter. Detailed information on this topic can be had from astrological works and those on *Ratna śāstra.*

The process of *māraṇa* essentially involves exposing the metal, etc. to the effect of the heat of fire. In other words this is a process of calcination. But some of these gems having cooling properties work better and produce potent therapeutic effects when used in the form of *piṣṭī* which does not involve exposure to heat. To make this gem digestible, absorbable and assimilable it is reduced to a fine powder form by grinding with rose-water or sandal-wood oil. Some of these gems and jewels are used in both the forms, viz., *piṣṭī* and *bhasma.*

Some animals and vegetable products are toxic by nature. To make them free from toxicity and to make them easily digestible, absorbable and assimilable, these are subjected to the process of *śodhana* and *māraṇa*. It is because of this that these vegetable and animal products are included within the scope of *rasa śāstra.* The processing of animal and vegetable products is described in the 8th and 9th chapters respectively.

Appendix-I elaborates technical terms used in *Rasa śāstra.* Some of these terms are used in this text and others are often used in other texts on this subject. Acquaintance with these terms is necessary for those interested in further study on this topic.

Appendix-II provides illustrated description of various equipments and implements commonly used in the processing of mercury and other metals as well as minerals.

The author had the good fortune to be a student of Prof. Vasudev M. Dwivedi at the Post Graduate Training Centre in Ayurveda at Jamnagar. Prof. Dwivedi has since retired from service. In spite of his advanced age, his mission for service to the suffering humanity through *rasa śāstra* is ceaselessly continuing. His devotion to alleviate the miseries of the suffering humanity inspired the author to undertake this work. The author is highly indebted to Prof. Dwivedi. For the preparation of this work Vaidya Lalitesh Kashyap, B.I.M.S., Ph.D., Superintendent of the CGHS Ayurvedic Hospital, New Delhi; Ku. Kanchan Gupta, M.A. (Sanskrit) and Shri Pradipta Kumar Dash were of constant help. Their help is thankfully acknowledged.

This work, I hope, will be useful to the students, teachers and research workers in ayurveda in general and *rasa śāstra* in particular in India and abroad. This provides a vast unexplored field for research to scientists.

BHAGWAN DASH

INTRODUCTION

Drugs used in Ayurveda can be broadly classified into three categories, viz., (a) vegetable products, (b) animal products, and (c) metals and minerals. In the Vedic literature and in ayurvedic classics, mostly vegetable drugs were prescribed for the treatment of different categories of ailments. Very few animal products and still fewer metals and minerals are described in those texts. Metals described in these works include iron, copper, gold, lead, tin, silver and copper pyrite. They were meant for both external and internal uses. In ayurvedic classics, mercury is also prescribed for external use. Metals for internal use were processed by impregnating with different kinds of decoctions as well as the juice of herbs, and thereafter, by drying in sun or shade. These metals were then reduced to a fine powder form by grinding in a mortar and pestle, and administered to the patient either alone or in combination with several other drugs. Making a *bhasma* or calcined powder of these metals was not very popular among the physicians of those days.

During the fifth century B.C. and thereafter, the important branch of Ayurveda namely *śalya tantra* was viewed as a form of *hiṃsā* or violence. *Ahiṃsā* or non-violence was the cardinal rule of the religion prevalent in those days. The religion which was adopted by the rulers and subjects alike, discouraged the practice of surgery and it was almost legally banned. This created a new problem. Some surgical conditions were, no doubt, amenable to the conventional remedies, mostly of vegetable products which were used in the practice at that time. Some special therapies like *pañca karma* which include emetic therapy (*vamana karma*), purgation therapy (*virecana karma*), medicated enema therapies (*nirūha* and *anuvāsana karmas*) and inhalation therapy (*nasya karma*) took care of some of these obstinate surgical conditions. But the practice of these therapies were also discouraged and later banned in the areas influenced by those religious leaders. At that time, physicians as well as other research workers took upon themselves the responsibility of developing medicines for the treatment of these obstinate surgical conditions and otherwise incurable diseases.

In the forefront of this adventure were the Buddhist monks. Compassion for all living beings was an essential part for their teaching and practice. Medical care was one of their esteemed methods for the propagation of religion. Above all, it is the propounders and followers of Buddhism who banned or discouraged the *śalya tantra* or surgery and the practice of *pañca karma* therapies. Therefore, they endeavoured to find alternatives for curing these obstinate surgical conditions. This provided an impetus to the progress of *Rasa śāstra* or the science dealing with therapeutic use of mercury and other metals. As a by-product, the science dealing with the transmutation of base metals into noble metals like gold with the help of processed mercury also received impetus. *Nāgārjuna*, the Bhuddhist philosopher and propounder of the *mādhyamika* sect of Buddhism was in the forefront of these physicians. Notwithstanding the controversy regarding the identity and period of *Nāgārjuna*, it can be safely stated that metals were processed and extensively used therapeutically in *bhasma* form prior to 3rd century A.D. Books composed on this subject by *Nāgārjuna* are mostly not available. Some books, authorship of which is attributed to *Nāgārjuna*, appear to be later compositions. Descriptive texts, now available on *Rasa śāstra*, were mostly composed during 8th century A.D. and thereafter.

Superiority of Mineral Drugs

In addition to curing obstinate and otherwise incurable conditions, mineral drugs were also used for the treatment of common diseases because of advantages which are summarised in the verse given below:

अल्पमात्रोपयोगित्वात् अरुचेरप्रसङ्गतः।
क्षिप्रमारोग्यदायित्वात् औषधेभ्योऽधिको रसः।।

"Mineral remedies are therapeutically effective even when adminstered only in a small dose (unlike vegetable products which are generally required to be administered in a much larger dose). These mineral products are not unpalatable (unlike some of the vegetable remedies which are sometimes very unpalatable because of bitter, astringent and pungent tastes). Mineral products produce their therapeutic effects instantaneously (unlike vegetable products which take longer time because they have to pass through the process of digestion and metabolism before they become therapeutically active)".

In view of the above, treatment with metallic and mineral preparations was considered to be superior in comparison to treatment with vegetable drugs and surgical therapies. It is said :

आसुरी मानुषी दैवी चिकित्सा त्रिविधा मता।
शस्त्रैः कषायैः लोहाद्यैः क्रमेणान्त्याः सुपूजिताः।।

"Therapies are of three categories, viz., *āsurī* (demoniac) which includes surgical therapies, (2) *mānuṣī* (human) which is performed by the use of decoctions, etc. of vegetable drugs, and (3) *daivī* (divine) which is performed by the administration of metallic and mineral preparations. The succeeding ones are superior to the preceding categories of therapies."

Distinctive Features

Ayurvedic concepts of drug composition and drug action are equally applicable to both the drugs of vegetable origin and metallic as well as mineral drugs. All these ingredients possess *rasa* (taste), *guṇa* (attributes), *vīrya* (potency), *vipāka* (taste which emerges after digestion) and *prabhāva* (specific action). All of them are composed of five *mahābhūtas*, viz. *pṛthvī, ap, tejas, vāyu* and *ākāśa*. In spite of this, there are several distinctive features because of the specific nature of the permutation and combination of these five *mahābhūtas* or basic elements in the composition of these drugs. In the ingredients of diet, *rasa* or taste is exceedingly manifested and the *vīrya* is in a latent form. In the vegetable drugs including animal products (notwithstanding exceptions), *rasa* (taste) is less manifested and *vīrya* is exceedingly manifested. In metallic and mineral products, *rasa* is latent whereas the *vīrya* or the protency is exceedingly potent. Therefore, therapeutically, metallic and mineral drugs are more useful than the vegetable and animal products.

Purpose of Processing

As has been mentioned before, during the classical age, metals and minerals were impregnated with decoctions, and juice of various types of vegetable drugs, and then reduced to a state of fine particle by grinding. During the later period, this technique of processing metals and minerals reached a very high stage of sophistication and scientific accuracy. For any drug to be therapeutically effective, it is necessary that it should be assimilated specially by the affected tissues. Metals and minerals, according to *mahābhautika* composition have a different structure than the tissue elements of the body. If these are used in raw form or even in unprocessed powder form, they will not be digested, absorbed, metabolised and assimilated to the tissue cells of the body. Thus, they will be therapeutically ineffective. On the other hand, these heterogeneous drugs are likely to produce serious toxic effect in the body. To make them non-toxic, to make them easily digestible and absorbable, to make them suitable for metabolic changes and assimilable by the tissue cells, and to make them therapeutically potent, several methods for processing have been prescribed. Depending upon the nature of the metal or mineral, they are first of all cleaned of their physical and chemical impurities and then triturated with the juice or decoctions of drugs. This impregnation or trituration loosens the molecular cohesiveness and helps the metal to break into fine particles during the subsequent processing. This also neutralises the toxic effects and makes the metal easily digestible and assimilable. The vegetable drugs which are used in the form of decoction or juice have their own therapeutic effects which are imparted to these metals during processing. Thereafter, the metal is dried and the moisture portion is taken out. These are made into small lumps and kept inside two earthen plates (*śarāva*). The borders of these two earthen plates containing lumps of metallic paste are kept together face to face and sealed with the help of seven layers of mud-smeared cloth. These earthen plates are kept exposed to sun till they are completely dried. These are then kept in a pit covered with the required number of cow-dung-cakes and ignited. Depending upon the heat requirement of each metal, the size of the pit and the number of cow-dung-cakes to be used vary. Then it is allowed to cool of its own and the earthen plates are removed from the heap of cow-dung ash. The seal is, thereafter, carefully, removed and metallic lumps are taken out for subsequent processing. Depending upon the nature of the metal and the disease for which they are meant to be used, the process is repeated for several times.

The first part of this processing with decoction, juice, etc. is called *śodhana* (lit. purification) and the latter part of this processing is called *māraṇa* (lit. killing) or reducing metal to a fine state of division while changing its physical and chemical nature.

The above mentioned methods vary from one metal to the other. Details of these methods will be described in respective sections.

Deha Siddhi and Lauha Siddhi

Metals and minerals including mercury are generally used in ayurveda for the treatment of simple as well as obstinate diseases. These are also used to prevent the occurrence of several categories of disease. The most important use of metal and mineral in ayurveda is for rejuvenation (*rasāyana*) which leads to the preservation and promotion of positive health. These drugs can be used by young and old people alike. In both, these drugs help in the maintenance and promotion of their positive health.

Concept of Health

Health according to ayurveda is not merely a condition of freedom from disease. According to Suśruta :

समदोषः समाग्निश्च समधातुमलक्रियः।
प्रसन्नात्मेन्द्रियमनाः स्वस्थ इत्यभिधीयते।।

[*Suśruta* : *Sūtra* 15:40]

"A person having equipoise of *doṣas* (factors controlling physiological activities of the body), *agnis* (factors responsible for digestion and metabolism), *dhātus* (tissue elements), *malas* (excreta) and *kriyā* (physical and mental activities), and a person who is possessed of spiritual, sensual and mental happiness is called a healthy person (*svastha*)".

Thus, the dimension of the concept to health in ayurveda is very wide. It is not only the physical fitness but the spiritual, sensual and psychological well-being which are considered to be the *sine qua non* for the health of an individual. This holistic concept of positive health is the unique feature of the ayurveda. Death after birth is inevitable. But the person should live a full span of life with his vision, hearing power and other sensual faculties intact. The death should be painless. This is what ayurveda stands for, and this is the purpose of *rasāyana* or rejuvenation therapy which is the most important branch of ayurveda. For this purpose, metals and minerals, in general, and mercury in particular, are used after exposing them to the prescribed methods of processing. In the parallel of *Rasa śāstra*, this is called *deha siddhi* or attainment of perfect health.

Aim of Rasāyana Therapy

The term *deha* is generally translated as the 'physique'. But in ayurveda, the concept of *deha* is much more subtle. It has five layers, viz. (1) *annamaya kośa* or the physical body which is nourished by the end-products of food and drinks, (2) *prāṇamaya kośa* or the layer of the body which sustains *prāṇa* or life force, (3) *manomaya kośa* or the layer of the body which is responsible for all psychic activities, (4) *vijñānamaya kośa* or the layer of the individual which is responsible for all intellectual activities, and (5) *ānandamaya kośa* or the layer of the individual which is responsible for all spiritual activities and where the individual enjoys eternal bliss. The *rasāyana* or rejuvenation therapy is meant to provide the required nourishment to all these five layers of the individual and not merely to the physical body.

Alchemical Achievements

The other aspect of the *rasa śāstra* is called *lauha siddhi* or the attainment of perfection in preparing noble metals like gold and silver from ordinary metals with the help of processed mercury. This important aspect of *rasa śāstra* is, no doubt, described in several ayurvedic texts. But the practice of this science is limited only to a few highly adept saints. The technique of preparing gold with the help of processed mercury is so exciting and so lucrative that there is every possibility of undesirable persons taking advantage of this knowledge and amassing wealth for themselves which in turn may be utilised to the detriment of the society. Nāgārjuna, the important propounder of *rasa śāstra* said :

सिद्धे रसे करिष्यामि निर्दारिद्र्यमिदं जगत् ।

"I shall make the entire world free from poverty by my attainments in processing of mercury with perfection."

For the above mentioned purpose, mercury has to undergo 18 stages of processing (*aṣṭādaśa saṃskāras*). During this step by step processing, the *bīja* (lit. seed) is prepared. This, in small quantity, has to be added to a large quantity of ordinary mercury or other base metal and heated with cow-dung-cakes by which the ordinary mercury is changed into gold. This may appear to be quaint. Of course, the physicist can perform this by bombarding the molecule of mercury which is, according to the atomic table, nearer to gold. But this process involves enormous expenditure and highly sophisticated equipments and experienced scientists. What is done in ayurveda is, no doubt, kept secret but the method is much more simple. An inscribed evidence of one such recent demonstration of this achievement is available in two mable plaques fixed in the wall of the *yajña vedī* (altar for fire sacrifice ceremony) behind the *Lakṣmī Nārāyaṇa* temple (also known as *Biralā* temple) in Delhi. It is written in Hindi and the English translation of this informative statement is given below :

"In the month of *Caitra* (name of the month according to the Hindu calender corresponding to March-April) of the *Vikrama Saṃvat* 1999 (1942 A.D.), one Śrī Kṛṣṇa Lāla Śarmā, Rasa Vaidya Śāstrī, originally hailing from Pubjab came from Ṛṣikeśa to Delhi to demonstrate the practical method of preparing gold out of mercury. On this occasion, the secretary of Mahātmā Gāndhī, Śrī Mahādeva Desāī, Gosvāmī Gaṇeśa Datta and Śrī Jugala Kiśora Biralā (the noted industrialist of India) were present. In front of them, 200 *tolās* or 2½ seers (1 *tolā* is approximately 12 Grams) of mercury was mixed with one *tolā* of the powder of a drug (identity undisclosed) and the whole thing was kept over fire for half an hour. Thereafter, the mercury became gold. This process was repeated, and as such 18 seers of gold was prepared."

Again in another plaque in the same place, the statement is as follows :

"On the first day of *śukla pakṣa* (bright fortnight) in the month of *Jyeṣṭha* (name of a month according to Hindu calender corresponding to May-June) of Saṃvat 1998 i.e. 27th May, 1941, Pt. Kṛṣṇa Lāla Śarmā in our presence (names of these persons are given below) prepared one *tolā* of gold from out of one *tolā* of mercury in Birala House, New Delhi. The mercury was kept inside a fruit of *rīṭhā* (bot. *Sapindus trifoliatus* Linn.). Inside this, a white powder of some herb and a yellow powder which were perhaps one or one and half *rattī* (one *rattī* is equal to 125 mg.) in weight were added. Thereafter, the fruit of *rīṭhā* was smeared with mud and kept over fire for about 45 minutes. During that process, the fire was made stronger with the help of a fan. When the charcoal after ignition became ash, water was sprinkled over it. From inside the fruit which originally contained mercury, gold came out. In weight, the gold was 1 to 2 *rattis* less than one *tolā* (originally used). It was pure gold. We could not ascertain the nature as well as the identity of both the powders which were added to the mercury were not disclosed to us. During the whole experiment, Pt. Kṛṣṇa Lāla was standing about 10 to 15 ft. away from us (site of performance). During this time Śrī Amṛta Lāla V. Ṭhakkara (Chief Secretary, *Akhil Bhāratīya Sevaka Saṅgha*), Śrī Gosvāmī

Gaṇeśa Dattajī (of Lahore), Secretary of Birla Mill in Delhi Śrī Khemakā, Chief Engineer Mr. Wilson and Śrī Viyogī Hari were present. We were all surprised to witness this performance. Seth Śrīmān Jugala Kiśora Biralā was kind enough to show us this performance.

Signed : (1) Amṛta Lāla V. Ṭhakkara

(2) Sītā Rāma Khemakā

(3) Viyogī Hari

Mārgaśīrṣa Kṛṣṇa 5, *Saṃvat* 2000, Delhi (This was perhaps the date of installation of the plaque).

Late Pt. Kṛṣṇa Lāla Śarmā, Rasa Vaidya Śāstrī learnt this technique from a saint named Nārāyaṇa Svāmī. But in the absence of a suitable disciple, according to him, he did not teach this technique to any body."

In addition to these written evidences, several other incidents of preparing gold out of mercury are described by people who are dependable and who vouch to have seen the technique themselves. In fact, to pursue scientific research into this technique, the Government of India in the Ministry of Health gave a token financial assistance to one of the disciples of Pt. Kṛṣṇa Lāla Śāstrī. Unfortunately, after starting the research work the saint who was living in Hardvāra died.

The above incidents have been described only to highlight that the technique of *lauha siddhi* (preparation of gold out of mercury) is not merely a myth but is factually correct. The technique is kept a well guarded secret to prevent its misuse by anti-social elements.

The earliest and most authentic record relating to the knowledge *lauha siddhi* i.e. transmutation of base metals or ordinary mercury into gold is found in the *Artha śāstra* (treatise on polity) of Kauṭilya or Cāṇakya, who was the well known Prime Minister of the Maurya King Candra Gupta during 4th century B.C. (1600 B.C. according to some historians). He has described, among others, a type of gold which is artificially prepared, obviously referring to the method of alchemy narrated above.

CHAPTER I

HISTORICAL BACKGROUND OF RASA ŚĀSTRA

Historical Background

The *Vedas* are the oldest repository of human knowledge. Ayurveda is one of the *upavedas* of or subsidiaries to the *Vedas*. Therefore, all topics including *Rasa śāstra* or Alchemy described in ayurveda are considered to be derived from the *Vedas*. The *Ṛkveda* describes iron in the context of the preparation of an artificial leg. The *Yajur veda* in the form of a prayer invokes the blessings of metals like iron, lead, tin and gold, among others, to bestow good health and longevity. The *Atharva veda* has classified treatment (*cikitsā*) into four categories, viz. (1) *ātharvaṇī*, (2) *āṅgirasī*, (3) *daivī*, and (4) *manuṣyajā*. The third variety i.e. *daivī cikitsā* has been explained in the subsequent alchemical texts to be dealing with metallic including mercurial preparations for the preservations as well as promotion of positive health and for prevention as well as cure of diseases. Presence of metals like iron in different tissues of the body has been described in one of the *mantras* (incantations) of the *Atharvaveda* and in this, *trapu bhasma*, i.e., tin in *bhasma* or calcined form is mentioned. This indicates that metals were being reduced to *bhasma* form at that time.

Several ayurvedic classics were composed thereafter. Unfortunately, most of them are not available now. We know about them only from the quotations taken from these works and reference made to them in subsequent books. The extant ayurvedic classics were composed prior to 7th century B.C.

Caraka[1] has classified drugs into three categories viz. (1) vegetable

1. According to some historians *Caraka saṃhitā* was composed during 13th century B.C.

products, (2) animal products, and (3) metals including minerals. The third category includes gold, iron-rust, copper, iron, tin, silver, lead, *sikatās* (different types of sand), *sudhā* (different calcium compounds), realgar, orpiment, gems and jewels, salts, red ochre and *añjana* (antimony). These metals are prescribed for both internal and external uses. Caraka has also prescribed mercury, sulphur and copper pyrite for internal use. Metals and minerals were impregnated with different kinds of decoctions and juice of herbs and dried in sun or shade. Thereafter, these metals were reduced to a fine powder form by grinding in a mortar and pestle and administered to the patient either alone or in combination with several other drugs.

Suśruta saṃhitā, which was also composed prior to 7th century B.C.[2], has described metals and minerals like gold, silver, copper, bell metal, tin, lead, iron and rust of iron for medicinal purposes. Mercury and sulphur are also described as external medicaments.

Even though metals and minerals were used both externally and internally for the preservation as well as promotion of positive health and prevention and cure of diseases, a significant reference to alchemy is made only in the *Arthaśāstra* of Kauṭilya during the 4th century B.C.[3] As a corollary to polity, this work described different types of metals, gems and jewels. One variety of gold described there is *Rasa viddha suvarṇa* i.e. gold prepared by transmutation of base metals with the help of mercury. This shows that even prior to his time, this type of gold was available in the market and people knew the techniques of conversion of base metals into noble metals with the help of mercury.

The third century witnessed another significant development in the field of ayurveda. *Caraka saṃhitā* and *Suśruta saṃhitā* were not available in their original form. Texts of these classics, which were then extant, were in a completely mutilated form and interpolated often by persons not entitled to do so. This invited attention of Vāgbhaṭa who prepared two works by compiling material from the then available works. He was a saivaite in the prime of his life but was defeated by Buddhists in a religious debate. According to the predetermined terms of the debate he was destined to death. But his life was saved and he was asked to complete his medical works viz. *Aṣṭāṅga hṛdaya* and *Aṣṭāṅga saṅgraha.* In these two works, several metals and minerals are mentioned to be used as remedies. Since these are based on earlier classics, description of metals and minerals was not given more importance than what it received in earlier classics. Following the footstep of his coreligious

2. According to some historians it was composed during 14th century B.C.
3. According to some historians it was composed during 16th century B.C.

leaders like Nāgārjuna, he, however, wrote a separate text on ayurveda dealing with *Rasa śāstra.* This text was called *Rasa ratna samuccaya.* Some historians consider it to be a latter work (13th to 15th cent. A.D.) and by a different Vāgbhaṭa which is not supported by enough internal and external evidences.

In 9th century A.D., Govinda Bhagavatpāda, the preceptor (*Guru*) of Śaṅkarācārya, the illustrious propounder of *Advaita vedānta,* composed *Rasa hṛdaya tantra* which provides elaborate description of the processing of mercury both for *loha siddhi* (preparing gold, etc., out of base metals) and *deha siddhi* (making the body free from ageing process and diseases leading to the state of *jīvan mukti*). During this century Tiṣṭācārya wrote *Cikitsā kalikā* where some metallic preparations in *bhasma* form were described for the treatment of diseases.

Tenth and eleventh centuries witnessed a different approach to the composition of ayurvedic works. Vṛnda Mādhava (10th century A.D.) supplemented the classical methods of treatment of diseases with metallic and mineral preparations and described the outline of their processing as well as preparation of *bhasma.* Cakrapāṇi (11th century A.D.), the eminent commentator of *Caraka saṃhitā* and *Suśruta saṃhitā,* in his work, also included metallic and mineral preparations for the treatment of diseases.

During 12th century A.D., following the footsteps of Govinda Bhagavatpāda, and in the form of a dialogue, another work called *Rasārṇava tantra* was composed. It is a work of *Śaiva sampradāya* (saivaite sect) and the author preferred to remain anonymous.

In this century, Siddha Nitya Nātha also composed his work called *Rasa ratnākara* dealing both with *deha siddhi* and *lauha siddhi.* He belonged to *Nātha* sect. *Rasendra cūḍāmaṇi* of Somadeva was also composed during this century.

During 13th century A.D. two important works on alchemy were composed. These are (1) *Rasa prakāśa sudhākara* by Yaśodhara, and (2) *Rasa sāra* by Govindācārya. Both of them deal with both *deha siddhi* and *lauha siddhi.*

Ḍhuṇḍuka Nātha, a saint of Saivaite sect composed *Rasendra cintāmaṇi* during 14th cent. A.D. During this century another Saivaite saint Gopāla Kṛṣṇa Bhaṭṭa composed *Rasendra sāra saṅgraha* which is mostly a compilation of earlier works. Devadatta's *Dhātu ratna mālā* also belongs to this century. The philosophical background of *jīvan mukti* (salvation while the individual is alive) was explained by Mādhavācārya during this century in his *Sarva darśana saṅgraha.* A separate section of this work called *Raseśvara darśana* deals with this topic.

In 15th century A.D., Śārṅgadhara composed his work *Śārṅgadhara saṃhitā* dealing with various aspects of ayurveda. While describing the treatment of diseases, he had followed, earlier physicians like Vṛnda as well as Cakrapāṇi, and along with classical recipes, mercurial and metallic preparations were described. Rāmarāja, the son of Ratna pāla composed *Rasa ratna pradīpa* and Bindu composed his *Rasa paddhati* during this century.

Sixteenth century witnessed several important activities in this field of *Rasa Śāstra* or alchemy perhaps because of the settled political condition that was prevailing then in India. Rāmakṛṣṇa Bhaṭṭa composed *Rasendra kalpa druma*. Jñāna Candra composed *Rasa kaumudī* and Cūḍāmaṇi Miśra composed *Rasa Kāma dhenu*—all dealing with mercury and other metals for both *deha siddhi* and *lauha siddhi*. Ṭoḍaramalla, the Minister of the Moghul King Akbar, composed his encyclopaedic work *Ayurveda Saukhya* in the *Ṭoḍarānanda* Series. This compilation work deals with basic principles, materia medica and diagnosis as well as treatment of diseases. Several chapters of this work are devoted to *Rasa śāstra*, and for the treatment of diseases several mercurial and metallic preparations are prescribed. (See Nineth Vol. of Ṭoḍarānanda Series-Iatro-Chemistry in Ayurveda, by the same author; published by Concept Publishing Company.)

Prāṇanātha's *Rasa pradīpa* and Kāyastha Cāmuṇḍa's *Rasa saṅketa kalikā* were also composed in the 16th century A.D. *Rasa pradīpa* described the preparation of *Rasa karpūra* for the treatment of syphilis and several pain-killers were described by adding opium and nux-vomica to mercury and sulphur in this century. Bhāva Miśra in his *Bhāva prakāśa* included several metallic preparations for the treatment of diseases.

In the 17th century A.D., *Dhātu kriyā* or *Dhātu mañjarī* was composed in the form of a dialogue between Śiva and Pārvatī on the lines of *Rasārṇava tantra*. The author of this work had preferred to remain anonymous. Bhikṣu Mayūra Pāda composed *Yoga ratnākara* during this century. In this work diagnosis and treatment of diseases are described. For the treatment, many metallic and mercurial compounds along with tobacco and *copacīnī* (*Smilex china* Linn.) are prescribed. *Āyurveda prakāśa* of Mādhava Upādhyāya is another important work composed during this period. It deals with the processing of mercury and other metals both for *deha siddhi* and *lauha siddhi*.

Bhaiṣajya ratnāvalī of Govinda Dāsa (18th century A.D.), *Bṛhat rasarāja sundara* of Dattarāma Caube (19th century) and *Rasa taraṅgiṇī* of Sadānanda Śarmā (20th century) provide extensive description of the use of mercurial and metallic preparations in the treatment of diseases. In 20th century, several other works were composed on *Rasa Śāstra*. These are *Rasāyana sāra* of Śyāma Sundarācārya, *Rasa jalanidhi* of Bhūdeva Mukhopādhyāya, *Pārada saṃhitā* of Nirañjana Prasāda Gupta, *Pārada vijñānīyam* of Vāsudeva Mūlaśaṅkara Dvivedī, *Rasa rāja mahodadhi* of Gaurī Śaṅkara Tripāṭhī, *Rasa yoga sāgara* of Hari Prapanna Śarmā, *Rasoddhāra tantra* of Jīvarāma Kālidāsa Śāstrī, *Rasa tantra sāra vā Siddha prayoga saṅgraha* of Svāmī Kṛṣṇānanda and *Rasāmṛta* of Yādavajī Trikamajī Ācārya. Efforts were made to revive *Rasa Śāstra* which was gradually going out of practice. Śyāma Sundarācārya and Bhūdeva Mukhopādhyāya claimed their personal experience that during *jāraṇa saṃskāra*, mercury digests and assimilates gold without any increase in weight. It is very difficult to say if they personally performed *lauha siddhi* (transmutation of base metals into noble metals with the help of processed mercury) or not, because this is usually kept secret in view of professional ethics and for fear of persecution by the rulers of the country. Vāsudeva Mulaśankara Dvivedī and Nirañjana Prasāda Gupta have furnished experimental data which were collected by them during the *saṃskāra* (processing) of mercury.

In the above, only important works are described. Several other works were composed on *Rasa Śāstra* in the past and most of them are lost to us. Their existence is known only from quotations taken from these works by subsequent authors. Most of the original works deal with both *deha siddhi* and *lauha siddhi*--*deha siddhi* emphasising upon *sadeha mukti* (attaining the state of salvation while alive), preservation as well as promotion of positive health and cure of obstinate diseases.

CHAPTER II

PHYSICO-CHEMICAL AND PHILOSOPHICAL CONCEPTS

PHYSICO-CHEMICAL CONCEPTS OF AYURVEDA

To correctly appreciate the scientific nature of *Rasa Śāstra* in ayurveda, it is necessary to be acquainted with its fundamentals specially with reference to physical and chemical concepts. So far as the creation of the universe and evolution of different categories of matter in general and metals in particular are concerned, ayurveda follows the physical theories of the *Sāṅkhya* and *Yoga*. The *Nyāya* and *Vaiśeṣika* systems are adopted in ayurveda with reference to the methodology of examination, mechanics, physics as well as chemistry. When ayurveda deals with transmigration of soul and concepts of salvation and the *saṃskāras* (impressions of the past life) which produce certain types of diseases, it is the *Vedānta* philosophy, in addition to the above, which is given primary importance.

According to the *Sāṅkhya* system, the manifested world is traced back to an unmanifested ground which is called *Prakṛti* or Primordial Matter Stuff. This *Prakṛti* is formless, undifferentiated, limitless and ubiquitous, indestructible and undecaying, ungrounded and uncontrolled, without beginning and without end. Eventhough it is conceived as a unity, this is merely an abstraction. It is in reality an undifferentiated manifold and indeterminate infinite continuum of infinitesimal Reals. These Reals are called *guṇas* and they are classified into three categories, viz. (1) *sattva* or essence, which manifests itself in a phenomenon, and which is characterised by this tendency to manifestation; it serves as the medium for the reflection of Intelligence and Consciousness; (2) *rajas* or energy is efficient in a phenomenon and is characterised by the tendency to work and to overcome resistance; and (3) *tamas* or inertia (mass) which counteracts the tendency of *rajas* to do work, and of *sattva* to conscious manifestation.

Thus, the ultimate reality of this universe are (1) *sattva* or essence or conscious factor, (2) *rajas* or energy, and (3) *tamas* or inertia characterised by mass. These *guṇas* or attributes are Reals and substantive entities but they are not independent entities. Therefore, they are not material, but they possess quantum and extensity. The very nature of energy or *rajas* is to do work, to overcome resistance and to produce motion. All energy is, therefore, ultimately kinetic in nature. The *sattva* or the consciousness manifests itself to intelligence and nothing exists without such manifestation in the universe of consciousness. It does not possess mass or gravity. It neither offers resistance nor does it work.

On the other hand, *tamas* representing mass, inertia or matter offers resistance to motion as well as to conscious reflection. The conscious element (*sattva*) and the matter stuff (*tamas*), by themselves, cannot do any work, and therefore, devoid of productivity in themselves. All works come from *rajas*, the principle of energy which overcomes resistance of matter and supplies even energy to the consciousness for the regulation or adaptation of its own manifestations.

These *guṇas* or attributes are always uniting, separating and uniting again. Everything in this world results from their peculiar arrangement and combinations. Though cooperating to produce the world of effects, these diverse tendencies of *guṇas* never coalesce with each other. Thus, in the phenomenal product, every energy is due to the element of *rajas*; all matter, resistance and stability are due to *tamas;* and all conscious manifestations are due to *sattva*.

STARTING OF COSMIC EVOLUTION

There is a condition of equilibrium or equipoise consisting of uniform diffusion of these Reals at the starting point of cosmic evolution. At this stage, the process of cosmic evolution is in a stage of standstill. The transcedental influence of the *Puruṣa* or the Absolute puts an end to this stage of arrest and initiates the process of creation. Evolution begins thereby with a disturbance in the state of this equilibrium. When the influence of the *Puruṣa* ends this state of arrest, the affinity which is inherent in *sattva*, *rajas* and *tamas* comes into play, breaks up the uniform diffusion and leads to unequal aggregation resulting in the relative preponderance of one or more of these *guṇas* over the other.

Thus, the process of evolution consists in the development of the differentiated within the undifferentiated, of the determinate within the indeterminate and of the coherent within the incoherent. This evolutionary series is subjected to a definite natural law. The order of succession is not from the whole to the part nor from parts to the whole but from relatively less differentiated, less determinate and less coherent whole to a more differentiated, more determinate and more coherent whole. This stage, represents a change from *avyakta* to *vyakta*.

The next stage of succession is the evolution of *Mahat* or Consciousness by differentiation and integration within the formless, characterless and inconceivable *Prakṛti* i.e. Primordial Matter Stuff.

The next step of evolution is bifurcation of this indeterminate stuff into Subject-series and Object-series. This process involves the manifestation of Ego or *Ahaṅkāra.* Predominance of *sattva* as well as *rajas* leads to the manifestation of Subject-series and the predominance of *rajas* as well as *tamas* results in the manifestation of Object-series. The Subject-series at a subsequent stage of evolution gets differentiated into *Indriyas* (sensory and motor stuff) and *Manas* or the Mind-stuff. The Object-series gives rise to the evolution of the *Tanmātrās* or *Sūkṣma bhūtas* which are determinate matter-stuff. These are the precursor agents for the evolution of atoms.

These *guṇas* or Reals, no doubt, assume infinite diversity of forms and powers, but they can neither be created nor destroyed. If the totality of the manifested as well as the unmanifested and the potential as well as the latent are taken into account, the mass (*tamas*), energy (*rajas*) and consciousness (*sattva*) remain constant. These are subjected to addition and substraction, growth and decay only because of changes of collocation and attainment of subsequent stage from the state of potential to the state of actual. In the course of evolution, these Reals conform to the natural law not only in the area of succession but also as regards to the appearance. This transformation in the process of cosmic evolution is constantly going on and it is not arrested even for a moment.

To explain the above mentioned phenomenon further, water remains still in a pond or water reservoir. If the boundary wall of this water reservoir is broken, then the water, on its own, moves to the field at a lower level without any body's effort. It continues to irrigate fields at a lower level provided water of the reservoir is at a higher level. It is the *Puruṣa* or the Absolute, Who is responsible for removing the obstruction and there His job ends, and the cosmic evolution continues.

EVOLUTION OF MATTER

As has been discussed above, because of predominance of *tamas* and *rajas*, the evolution of the Object-series takes place and the Subject-series is dominated by *rajas* and *sattva*. Before this, the *Prakṛti* in its successive stages of evolution upto the stage of *Ahaṅkāra* (Ego) is absolutely homogeneous and inert, and it is devoid of all physical and chemical characters except mass. This can neither be added nor subtracted, and this is neither created nor destroyed. During the subsequent step, however, transformations take place and the *tanmātrās* representing quantas of energy have attributes like penetrability (including vibrations), impact, radiation including heat, viscousity and cohesiveness. In intimate relation to these physical characters, these *tanmātrās* also possess the potentials of energy represented by sound, touch, colour, taste and smell. These potentials arise from the unequal distribution of the *tamas* or original mass-units in different proportions and collocations because of an unequal distribution of the *rajas* or original energy. But being subtle matter, these are devoid of peculiar forms which these potentials assume at a later stage of gross matter like *mahābhūtas* or atoms and molecules.

These *tanmātras* are infra-atomic particles charged with specific potential energy as has been discussed above. At a subsequent stage of evolution, the potential of sound stimulus is lodged in one class of particles or *tanmātras* possessing the physical energy of vibrations. They serve to form the radical of *ākāśa paramāṇu*. Then the potential of tactile stimulus lodged in another class of particles, which possess the physical energy of impact or mechanical pressure in addition to that of vibration serves to form the radical of *vāyu paramāṇu*. In the third stage, the class of *tanmātrās* having the potential of colour stimulus and charged with the energy of radiation (heat and light), in addition to those of impact and vibration, serve to form the radical of *tejas paramāṇu*. During the fourth stage, *tanmātrās* having taste stimulus and possessed with the energy of viscousity, in addition to those of radiation, impact and vibration, develop into the radical of *ap paramāṇu*. Lastly, the class of *tanmātrās* with the potential of smell stimulus and charged with the energy of cohesiveness in addition to those of viscousity, radiation, impact and vibration, serve to form the radical of *pṛthvī paramāṇu*.

There are diverse views about the process of creation of these *paramāṇus* from *tanmātrās*, but what has been stated above represents the ayurvedic concept according to which drug composition and drug action are explained.

EVOLUTION OF MAHĀBHŪTAS

The concept that is directly relevant to ayurvedic *Rasa Śāstra* and alchemy is the evolution of *mahābhūtas* from the *tanmātrās* and *paramāṇus* because it is these *mahābhūtas,* which in gross form, constitute metals. *Saṃskāras* or the specific methods prescribed for processing, aim at changing the *mahābhautika* composition of metals with a view to bringing *deha siddhi* and *lauha siddhi.* Aggregates of *paramāṇus,* keeping in view their structure, may be divided into two categories, viz. (1) those of which the parts are in intimate union of fusion being lost in the whole, and (2) mechanical aggregates or collocations of distinct and independent parts.

The former can be divided into two sub-categories viz., (1) the *bhūtas* and their isomeric modifications, and (2) chemical compounds. These chemical compounds (the latter group) may again be divided into two classes, viz. (i) those composed of atoms of the same *bhūta,* and (ii) those composed of atoms of different *bhūta* classes. The first kind leads to intimate union in which the isomeric atoms are attracted towards each other by a peculiar nature of energy and the second kind of contact between heterogeneous *bhūtas* begins with the liberation of energy which breaks up each of the *bhūtas* and taking particles of one as nucleus or radical, group particles of the remaining *paramāṇus* around these radicals in a comparatively free and unattached condition. In this case the molecule or *bhūta paramāṇu* which forms the radical becomes the material cause even if it is not predominant in the compound, and the remaining *paramāṇus,* which by their collocation give rise to the liberation of energy, are called the efficient causes. In addition to this transformation of the substance by isomeric or heterogeneous process, a number of other changes take place in the character, the modality and the state of substances due to unequal distribution of the force among the *guṇas* which are in themselves constant.

These *bhūtas* which are also called *sūkṣma bhūtas* then combine in different proportions with the radical as its material cause and other *bhūtas* as efficient cause to form *mahābhūtas.* Atoms and for that matter *sūkṣma bhūtas* cannot exist in this phenomenal universe in an uncombined form. Two of these *aṇus* (*paramāṇus*) combine to form a molecule which is called *dvyaṇuka.* Three of these *dvyaṇukas* combine to form a *tryaṇuka.* In this way, bigger and bigger *mahābhautika* molecules are formed. This process of combination of *paramāṇus* is the result of *parispanda* i.e. rotary or vibratory motion which is inherent in these *aṇus.*

Except *ākāśa,* all other *tanmātrās* have attributes of the previous ones in the subsequent ones. It is not possible to find in the phenomenal manifested world, *bhūtas* in pure form. What we find is actually a mixture of all the five *bhūtas.* The predominant one with manifested or unmanifested attributes form the radical and the remaining four form the subsidiary ingredients. This process is called *Pañcīkaraṇa* or the quintuplication.

All metals are basically dominated by *pṛthvī mahābhūta* characterised by cohesiveness. But in some of them as in mercury and gold, *tejas* corpuscles form the radical and the earth particles are dynamic. The metal mercury is chosen both for *deha siddhi* and *lauha siddhi* because in spite of *tejas* corpuscles as its radical and predomination of *pṛthvī* corpuscles as dynamic, it is relatively less cohesive, and therefore, by exposing it to different processes (*saṃskāras*) it is easily amenable to a change in its *bhautika* composition by which it can get assimilated into the body cells effectively as well as easily, and it can successfully penetrate into *mahābhautika* composition of base metals to transform them into a new compound of noble metals. This metal as such is ineffective but by subjecting it to different forms of processing (*saṃskāras*) adequate amount of energy inherent in its *paramāṇus* is liberated to effect such changes.

During the *saṃskāras* of mercury, it is either triturated or boiled with different types of herbal juices and organic acids over fire. Now it is necessary to examine the *modus operandi* of heat which is employed in different forms to bring about the changes in mercury. Juices of herbs including oils, fats and organic acids have the *paramāṇus* of *pṛthvī* which are dissolved or combined with the *paramāṇus* of *jala*. It is only when the *jala paramāṇu* congregates round the *pṛthvī paramāṇu* that dynamic contact produces peculiar characters like colour, taste and smell under the impact of *tejaṣ* corpuscle. Thereafter, under further impact they fall into groupings or collocation which determine the nature of the composite substance thus produced. All of them have *pṛthvī paramāṇu* as radical in dynamic collocation with *jala paramāṇu*.

MOLECULAR AND ATOMIC MOTIONS

Tanmātrās (quanta of energy), *paramāṇus* (atoms as conceived in ayurveda) and *mahābhūtas* (molecular entities as conceived in ayurveda) are in a constant state of motion which is called *parispanda*. The term *parispanda* means whirling, rotary, circling or vibratory motion. All action, operation or work are ultimately traced to this form of motion lodged in the atoms of substances. This rule applies to all substances in the universe including mercury and other metals. However, in comparison to other metals, this *parispanda* is exceedingly manifested in mercury inasmuch as in spite of its heavy weight, it is in normal state a liquid and exceedingly fickle. In view of this explicit manifestation of *parispanda*, it is amenable to changes at molecular, atomic and even *tanmātrika* levels which are essential for the creation for the type of energy required for both *deha siddhi* and *lauha siddhi*.

HEAT AND ITS MANIFESTATION

For bringing about physico-chemical changes in mercury and other metals, heat is invariably applied in different forms. Every atom, which itself is a mixture, has its own heat, and heat can also be applied from outside through sun rays and fire in the form of drying, boiling, burning, etc. When we burn fuel, it is the *tejas mahābhūta* or *tejas paramāṇu* which has remained latent in the exceedingly predominant *pṛthvī mahābhūta* that is made to manifest itself through the process of ignition.

Solar heat is the source of all the stores of heat required for chemical changes in the world. As it happens in the macro-cosmic level (the universe), the same thing happens in the micro-cosmic level i.e. individual. This *agni* or *tejas mahābhūta*, which is present inside the body and which comes from outside through food and drinks, is responsible for all phenomena associated with digestion and metabolism. Heat consists of indefinitely small particles which radiate in all directions rectilinearly with unconceivable velocity. The action of the heat takes place in three different ways. Heat particles may penetrate through the inter-atomic or inter-molecular space as in the case of conduction of heat. When water is kept in a pot which is a good conductor of heat, then these heat particles coming from below enter into the particles of water inside the pot without bringing any chemical or physical change in molecular collocation. The mechanism of conduction of heat in the present case is like the penetration of fluids through a porous body.

An alternative mode of action is that the particles of heat strike the atom or the molecule of the pot and stimulate the *tejas mahābhūta* or *tejas tanmātrā* inside those *paramāṇus*, which in turn induces similar changes in the next atom above it till it reaches the water where similar phenomenon takes place when water starts boiling. In the second method also the atoms or molecules of the pot do not undergo any change like decomposition, recomposition and alteration in collocation. The third alternative method is that the particles of heat strike the object in such a way so as to break up their grouping and transform the physico-chemical characters of the atoms, and may again recombine them all by means of continual impact with unconceivable velocity. This operation explains the process which takes place during chemical combination.

All these three modes of action are relevant in the context of *Rasa Śāstra* of ayurveda. When mercury is kept along with other medicines inside a pot and boiled, the first and second mechanisms become relevant for the heat to penetrate the pot and make the water as well as other ingredients inside the pot to boil. It is the third mechanism of heat which gradually brings about all the changes inside the mercury atom which after subsequent processing becomes suitable both for *deha siddhi* and *lauha siddhi*.

APPLICATION OF FORCE

Force can the applied as follows :

1. *Nodana* or continued pressure;
2. *Abhighāta* or impact; and
3. *Saṃskāra* or persistent tendency.

This third form of force is of two kinds viz. (1) *vega* (impressed motion or momentum) and (2) the tendency for the restoration of its original shape (*sthiti sthāpaka*). When mercury is triturated with the help of mortar and pestle all the three types of forces play their role. It is the weight of the pestle which produces the first type of force, is called *nodana* (continued pressure). The pressure is exercised over the pestle causes the second type of force, called *abhighāta* (impact). The motion in a body results from the combined motion of its particles. The pressure or impact produces mainly in an opposite direction the *vega* which is impressed upon the substance when the original direction gets changed. The pestle rebounding after initial impact illustrates such a change or direction in *vega* or motion. Thus, motions ultimately affect the *parispanda* or vibratory motion that is inherent inside the atoms to bring about a change in its energy components and to liberate energy with the help of heat that is employed both for *deha siddhi* and *lauha siddhi*. Drugs in the form of juices, decoctions or paste, which are added during these processes, facilitate the activities of heat for the liberation of this energy.

PHILOSOPHICAL BACKGROUND

The primary aim of *Rasa Śāstra* or Iatro-chemistry is not to convert base metals into noble metals. *Dhātu vedha saṃskāra*, which makes mercury potent to convert ordinary mercury or copper or tin into gold, is only a test to see that mercury is really potent enough to cause rejuvenation. In fact, wealth acquired by *dhātu vedha* or *lauha siddhi* is not supposed to be utilised for any personal benefit. It can be used only for charitable purposes, and if used for selfish purposes it is considered to be a sin and this may lead to several undesirable after effects. It is in view of this that most of the saints who are adepts in this science select disciples carefully and disclose them the exact process in confidence after properly assessing their mental and spiritual achievements. If suitable disciple is not available then they prefer not to teach any body and die with their knowledge. *Dhātu vedha* is only a method of testing the potency of mercury, and thereafter, it should be used for *deha siddhi* or the rejuvenation therapy.

Philosophical background of this science is called *Raseśvara darśana*. It belongs to *Māheśvara sampradāya* which has several subsects like *śaiva*, *pāśupata* and *bhairava*. The primary aim of this sect is to make the individual free from the process of ageing and to promote his longevity. Once this is achieved, with the additional help of various yogic methods, the person becomes capable of appreciating, understanding and realising the ultimate reality and, thus, he becomes the *jīvan mukta*. Most of the authors of *Rasa Śāstra* are, therefore, saints of great eminence. The ultimate aim of life, according to Indian tradition, is to attain happiness in this life and salvation thereafter.

Broadly speaking, Indian philosophers can be classified into two categories viz. (1) those who believe in ascertaining truth only by direct observation, and (2) those who believe in non-violence, etc., along with direct observation as the mode of ascertaining truth. Those belonging to the former group are called *Cārvākas* and others are called *Tārkikas*. *Tārkikas* are again of two types viz. *nāstikas* (who do not believe in the authority of the *Vedas* like Bauddhas and Jains) and *Āstikas* (those who believe in the authority of the *Vedas*). The *Āstikas* are again divided into two categories viz. *Saguṇātma vādī* (those who believe in the attributes of the Soul) and *Nirguṇātma vādī* (those who believe that the Soul is free from any attributes). These *Saguṇātma vādīs* are again divided into two categories viz. *Videha mukta vādī* (those who believe that salvation is possible only after death) and *Jīvan mukta vādī* (those who believe that one can attain salvation even while remaining alive).

These *Jīvan mukta vādīs* are the followers of *Raseśvara darśana*. By adopting various methods prescribed in different religious works one can attain salvation after his death. This is undoubtedly true but this is of little use to the person and to the society. According to the *Raseśvara darśana*, it is the body of the individual which is very important because through this body the individual can perform several activities for the development of his own soul, for the benefit of the society and for the realisation of the ultimate reality. If the body perishes, the individual becomes deprived of the vehicle through which he has to perform various religious rites; without the performance of religious rites there is no possibility of performing *yoga*; without the performance of *yoga* the mind cannot be controlled; and without the control of the mind realisation of the ultimate reality and salvation are impossible.

The body cells get destroyed at every moment, new body cells take their place and even more cells are produced for the growth. This anabolic process continues for some time till the person attains youth. Thereafter, there is a process of stagnation. Destruction of the body cells continues and the manufacture of new cells takes place in limited quantity which is sufficient to replace destroyed ones only. In old age this does not happen. There is more of destruction of body cells and much less of manufacture of new cells. Therefore, the individual succumbs to several diseases like bronchitis, asthma, arthritis, rheumatism, high blood pressure, heart disease, nervous disorders and digestive disorders. Gradually wrinkles appear in his body; his hair becomes grey; he loses eye-sight;his power of hearing diminishes and he loses his teeth. This nearly perishing body is also incapable of serving the purpose of a vehicle for the performance of religious rites and practice of *yoga* culminating in the control of the mind, realisation of the absolute self and salvation. Therefore, the person should not only have his body but he should have a healthy body, free from diseases and other complications of old age.

Not only long life or a healthy life is adequate for attaining salvation. Nor the control of mind is enough for this purpose. It is when both of them combine together i.e. when a controlled mind is located in a healthy and strong body, only then salvation could be achieved. The argument advanced against *jīvan mukta vāda* is that *jīvatva* (the process of living) and *muktatva* are two mutually opposite phenomenon. Both of them cannot be achieved simultaneously. This presumption is not correct. If *mukti* or salvation of the individual is expected as it is done by all the spiritual leaders then it is to be treated as an object of knowledge (*jñāna*). If it is an object of knowledge then there should be some body to appreciate or know about it (*jñātṛ*) and the best person to do that is the individual himself. Therefore, according to *Raseśvara darśana*, *jīvan mukti* is the only form of salvation which one should try to attain.

Processed mercury helps in bringing stability and endowing strength to the physique (*deha*) of the individual. This also helps in tuning of the mind to become free from worldly attachments, and this type of mind is capable of realisation of the Ultimate Reality which results in salvation. *Raseśvara darśana* is approved and adopted by all the spiritual leaders because of its unique features in dealing with the characteristics of the soul, characteristics of salvation and the relationship between the body and the soul. The great saint Govinda Bhagavatpāda in his reputed work, called *Rasa-hṛdaya tantra*, has summarised the state or *jīvan mukti* as follows :

तिष्ठन्त्यणिमादियुता विलसद्देहा मुदा सदानन्दाः।
ये ब्रह्मभावममृतं संप्राप्ताश्चैव कृतकृत्याः।।
भ्रूयुगमध्यगतं यच्छिखिविद्युन्निर्मलं जगद्भासि।
केषांचित्पुण्यकृतामुन्मीलति चिन्मयं ज्योतिः।।
परमानन्दैकमयं परमं ज्योतिः स्वभावमविकल्पम्।
विगलितसर्वक्लेशं ज्ञेयं शान्तं स्वयंवेद्यम्।।
तस्मिन्नाधाय मनः स्फुरदखिलं चिन्मयं जगत्पश्यन्।
उत्सन्नकर्मबन्धो ब्रह्मत्वमिहैव चाप्नोति।।
अस्तं हि यान्ति विषयाः प्राणान्तःकरणसंयोगात्।
स्फुरणं नेन्द्रियतमसां नातः स्फुरतश्च दुःखसुखे।।
रागद्वेषविमुक्ताः सत्याचारा नरा मृषारहिताः।
सर्वत्र निर्विशेषा भवन्ति चिद्ब्रह्मसंस्पर्शात्।।

[*Rasahṛdaya* 1 : 21-26]

"It is only in the virtuous ones, the flame full of consciousness appears between the two eye-brows which in appearance is like fire, *vidyut* (lightening) or sun. It is difficult to describe the nature of this excellent flame. It endows the person with eternal bliss and makes him free from all miseries. It is observable. It is peaceful and its attributes can be appreciated by the individual himself. The individual should concentrate his mind on this flame and the entire universe will appear before him like eternally vibrating consciousness. He becomes free from all types of attachments including those caused by the earlier actions of the present and past lives. He attains *Brahmatva* (characteristics of the Universal Soul) even in the present state of his life. All his desires get gradually diminished because of the combination of his *elan vitae* with his mind, intellect and soul. All vibrations of his senses stop and the mind does not undergo any change in happiness and miseries. He becomes free from attachments and envy. He practises only truth and becomes free from falsehood. Because of the contact of mind with the ultimate reality, he maintains equipoise in all circumstances. He is endowed with *aṣṭa siddhis* (eight excellent achievements like *aṇimā* (atomicity or subtility), etc. and while residing in the body enjoys eternal bliss. Those individuals who have attained this state of *Brahman* (unity with Universal Soul), which is like *amṛta* (ambrosia), are the real blessed ones."

Chapter III

RASA AND RASAŚĀLĀ

Definition

The branch of ayurveda dealing with processing and therapeutic use of metals, minerals and allied products is called the *Rasa śāstra. Śāstra* means 'knowledge' or 'science' and *rasa* means 'metals' and 'minerals' in general and 'mercury' in particular. According to the *Rasa ratna samuccaya* :

रसनात्सर्वधातूनां रस इत्यभिधीयते ।
जरारुङ्मृत्युनाशाय रस्यत वा रसो मतः ।।

[*Rasa ratna samuccaya* 1 : 76]

"Mercury has the power to assimilate (*rasanāt*) all the other metals because of which it is called *rasa.* In addition, it is effective (*rasyate*) in preventing and curing the process of ageing, pain and even death (untimely) for which it is called *rasa*".

These two definitions pertain to two different aspects of *siddhi*--the first one to *lauha siddhi* and the second one to *deha siddhi. Rasa* is a generic term which is applicable to all the metals including mercury. It also connotes mercury alone. For *deha siddhi*, mercury and other metals are used after appropriate processing, but for *lauha siddhi* only mercury is effective. For *lauha siddhi*, mercury has to undergo approximately 18 stages of processing which in the parallel of *rasa śāstra* are called *saṃskāras.* Details of these *saṃskāras* (stages of processing) will be discussed latter.

Classification

Metals and minerals are classified variously by different authors. Notwithstanding their dovetailing and the repetition under different categories the broad classification of metals and minerals is given below:

1. *Rasa*

In the present context this term specially pertains to mercury. Its several synonyms like *rasendra*, *sūta* and *pārada*--all these terms connote different aspects, viz. physical, chemical, physiological, therapeutic and spiritual aspects of this metal.

2. *Mahārasas (lit. Major Varieties of Rasa)*

These are *mākṣika* (Copper pyrite), *vimala* (Iron pyrite), *śilā jatu* (Mineral pitch or bitumen which is an exudate from a special type of stone), *Capala* (bismith), *rasaka* (a zinc ore), *sasyaka* (Copper sulphate), *hiṅgula* (Cinnabar), *śrotoñjana* (Antimony), *abhraka* (Mica), *rajavarta* (Lapis lazuli) and *vaikrānta* (Tourmaline).

3. *Uparasas (lit. Subsidiary Metals and Minerals)*

These are *gandhaka* (Sulphur), *haritāla* (Yellow arsenic or orpiment), *saurāṣṭrī* (Alum), *kāśīśa* (Iron sulphate), *gairika* (Red ochre) and *Kaṅkuṣṭha* (?).

4. *Sādhāraṇa Rasas (lit. Drugs Generally Used in the Processing of Mercury)*

These are *kampillaka* (it is a vegetable product; the botanical name of the plant is *Mallotus philippinensis* Muell-Arg.; the minute red glands and hair of the fruits of this plant are used in medicine), *gaurī pāṣāṇa* (White arsenic), *nava sāraka* (Ammonium chloride), *kapardaka* (cowrie-shell--this is an animal product), *vahni jāra* (Amber--this is an animal product), *giri sindūra* (Red lead) and *mṛddāra śṛṅga* (Litharge).

5. *Dhātus (Metals)*

These are *svarṇa* (Gold), *raupya* (Silver), *tāmra* (Copper), *vaṅga* (Tin), *yaśada* (Zinc), *nāga* (Lead) and *loha* (Iron).

6. *Upadhātus (Subsidiary Metals and Mineral Products)*

These are *svarṇa mākṣika* (Copper pyrite), *vimala* (Iron pyrite), *tuttha* (Copper sulphate), *kāṃsya* (Bronze), *pittala* (Bell metal), *sindūra* (Vermilion) and *śilā jatu* (Mineral pitch or bitumen which is an exudate from a special type of stone).

In addition to the above, *rasa śāstra* includes description, processing and therapeutic use of drugs belonging to the following categories :

1. *Ratnas* (gems and jewels);
2. *Uparatnas* (subsidiary gems and jewels);
3. *Sudhās* (calcium compounds);
4. *Lavaṇas* (salts);
5. *Kṣāras* (alkalies);
6. *Jāṅgama dravyas* (animal products);
7. *Viṣas* (vegetable products having acute toxic effects); and
8. *Upaviṣas* (vegetable products having less of toxicity).

RASAŚĀLĀ (PHARMACEUTICAL LABORATORY)

Before entering into the discussion relating to the selection and processing of the metals and minerals for therapeutic purposes, it is necessary to get acquainted about the selection of place and construction of the pharmaceutical laboratory and selection of teacher, students, physicians as well as helpers for this work. An outline of the same is provided below :

Construction

While selecting a place for the establishment of a pharmacy and during construction, following points should be kept in view :

1. It should be free from impediments—both man-made and providential;
2. Green and dried herbs should be available in the campus or nearby or they can be cultivated and stored inside;
3. It should look beautiful and be located near the sources of water like wells, ponds and rivers;
4. The area should be surrounded by a boundary wall;
5. The statue of *Rasa bhairava (Rasa liṅga)* should be located

in the eastern side;

6. In *agni koṇa* (south-east direction) fire-place, ovens, etc. required for cooking should be located;
7. Equipments for trituration, making paste, etc. should be located in the southern side;
8. *Nairṛtya koṇa* (place in the south-east direction) should be used for manufacturing and storing *yantras* (cooking equipments);
9. The place in western side should be used for washing;
10. Green herbs and freshly prepared medicines should be dried in the *vāyavya koṇa* (north-western direction);
11. The place in the northern side should be used for processing mercury and other metals as well as minerals;
12. *Bhasma* (processed fine powders of mercury, metals and minerals), tablets, medicated oils, medicated ghee, linctus, etc., should be stored in the house located in the *īśāna koṇa* (north-eastern direction).

Equipments and Raw Drugs

The following equipments and raw drugs which are frequently required should be stored in the pharmaceutical laboratory :

1. Pestles and mortars of different size and shape. These are made of either stone or iron or crystals;
2. Bottles, pots, cups, plates, utensils and jars made of glass, mud, wood as well as metals for storing raw drugs and finished products;
3. Equipments like forceps, spatula, spoon, knife, scissors, sieves, crucibles and *yantras* (for cooking);
4. Weighing machines and balances of different capacity and shape;
5. Different types of fuel like wood, cow-dung cake, coal, charcoal and husk; and
6. Mercury, other metals, minerals, drugs of vegetable origin, animal products, poisons of vegetable and animal origin, salts, alkalies, gems and jewels.

Pharmacy Assistants

Attendant to be employed in the pharmacy for assisting the physician in the processing and manufacture of various categories of drugs should have the following characteristics :

1. He should be energetic and enthusiastic to learn and assist the physician;
2. He should have physical and mental purity;
3. He should be brave, strong and careful;
4. He should be truthful, sincere and honest; and
5. He should take only wholesome food and regimens.

Teacher of Rasa śāstra

A teacher of *Rasa śāstra* should have the following characteristic features :

1. He should be of noble character and high morality and be compassionate, kind and truthful;
2. He should have attained perfection in the practice of *mantras*;
3. He should be a devotee of Lord Śiva;
4. He should have patience, courage and be in harmony with the laws of nature; and
5. He should be well versed in various aspects of *Rasa śāstra* - both the theory and the practice.

Suitable Students of Rasa Śāstra

Because of immense potentiality for being misused for materialistic and selfish gains which are to be strictly avoided, it is necessary to carefully examine the student before he is initiated to this branch of science. Such a student should have the following characteristic features:

1. He should be of noble character, high morality, expert in his traditional profession, respectful to teacher, brave, truthful, determined to acquire knowledge, obedient and free from laziness;
2. He should belong to a noble family, be clever and should be well versed in the theory and practice of other branches of ayurveda; and

3. He should be completely devoted to the teacher and his studies.

Unsuitable Students

Persons having the following characteristic features are not suitable for teaching :

1. Persons of bad character and conducts;
2. Persons borne in a low family;
3. Persons who are egoistic, thieves, deceptive and desirous of acquiring knowledge by any means;
4. Persons of unknown family lineage and conduct;
5. Persons who do not believe in the existence of God, sacred scriptures and life after death ; and
6. Persons who speak ill of the teacher.

Physicians for Rasaśālā

To help the teacher in day to day work, some physicians should be employed in the pharmacy and they should be as follows :

1. They should be specially interested in this branch of Ayurveda dealing with the processing of mercury, other metals, minerals, gems and jewels;
2. They should be acquainted with the identification and properties of drugs;
3. They should be acquainted with the explanation of different technical terms which often carry a secret implication; and
4. They should be acquainted with the name of drugs in different regional languages.

Amṛta Hasta Vaidya

Certain physical signs and mental attitude determine the superiority of the physician. When a medicine is touched by their hands, the effect becomes more. They are called '*Amṛta hasta*', i.e., one having nectar in the hand. These are as follows :

1. Auspicious signs like flag, jar, lotus, fish and bow in the palm; and
2. A line below the ring finger going downwards.

CHAPTER IV

PĀRADA (MERCURY)

SYNONYMS

Rasa, rasendra, sūta, raseśa, raseśvara, capala, rasa rāja and all the Sanskrit synonyms of Lord Śiva—these are the synonyms of mercury.

It is called *rasa* because it has the power to digest and assimilate other metals and minerals like mica. Since it is the most important in comparison to other metals and minerals, it is called *rasendra.* Since it produces *deha siddhi* and *lauha siddhi,* it is called *sūta.* Because of its fickleness it is called *capala.* Since it is the king among other metals and minerals it is called *rasa rāja.* It carries all the Sanskrit synonyms of Lord Śiva because it represents His essence. It is well known as *pārada* because it helps a person to achieve salvation.

Mercury or quick silver is the most important metal used in ayurveda both for *deha siddhi* (maintenance as well as promotion of positive health and prevention as well as cure of obstinate and otherwise incurable diseases) and *lauha siddhi* (alchemy or transmutation for ordinary metals into noble metals like gold and silver). This liquid metal is 13½ times heavier than water and gets evaporated when heated up to 357.25° centigrade. In colour, it is dazzling white and it is free from any smell or taste. It forms an amalgam with most of the metals except iron. Therefore, it should not be stored or processed in a vessel of copper, silver, bronze, etc. and should be stored and triturated only in containers of stone, glass mud, iron or enamel coated vessels. In view of its heavy weight, for alchemical processes, it is safer to keep it either in iron containers or in enamel vessels. Small quantities of this metal may, however, be stored in glass bottles.

According to ayurveda, mercury which is bluish in the centre and dazzling white outside is suitable for therapeutic use after processing. If it is smoky or pale or yellow in colour, it should not be used.

SOURCE

It is generally available near the volcanic hills. In the mines of Spain, it is available below 1600 ft., and in California at about 2200 ft. deep. In the mines of Almend in Spain and in California the output of mercury is maximum. Mercury is also available in Yugoslavia, Peru, Mexico, Italy, China and Australia. Its chief ore cinnabar is available in Afghanistan, Ireland, Burma and China. Other mercurial ores are available in South Africa, Australia, New Zealand, France, Germany, Hungary, Portugal and Japan.

MERCURY ORES

In mines, mercury is available in different forms as follows :

1. *Native Mercury*

In some mines this liquid metal is available as such, of course mixed with some impurities. Generally, they are obtained from certain pockets or caves inside these mines along with other metals.

2. *Mercurial Ores*

There are several compounds from which mercury is collected. The principal ore is cinnabar (HgS). Cinnabar is available in the mines in the form of Rhombohedral crystals, Hepatic cinnabar, Meta cinnabar, Coral ore, Steel ore and Brick ore.

EXTRACTION OF MERCURY FROM CINNABAR

Extraction of mercury from cinnabar has been described in several ancient ayurvedic texts like *Rasa sāra* (12th century A.D.), *Rasa ratnākara* (12th and 13th century A.D.), *Rasa ratna samuccaya* (13th century A.D.), *Rasa paddhati* (14th century A.D.), *Rasa prakāśa sudhākara* (13th or 14th century A.D.) and *Āyurveda prakāśa* (17th century A.D.). For extracting of mercury *Ūrdhva pātana yantra, Adhaḥ pātana yantra, Tiryak pātna yantra, Vidyādhara yantra* and *Ḍamaru yantra* are used. Details of these equipments are provided in App. II. This is considered to be free from any defect and according to some texts it can be used in ayurvedic medicines directly. This observation is, however, controversial.

Cinnabar is made to a powder. Then it is impregnated with lemon juice or the juice of the leaves of *nimba* (*Azadirachta indica* A. Juss) for three hours. This is then reduced to a fine state of division. Thereafter, mercury is extracted by keeping the paste in one of the above mentioned equipments.

DOṢAS OR DEFECTS IN MERCURY

Mercury as such is poisonous to the body cells. Like other metals and minerals, it is a foreign element, and when introduced into the body, there are reactions in tissue cells to throw it out. In addition, in the nature, pure mercury is seldom available. It is adulterated or contaminated with other elements which make this metal more poisonous for the body. Before mercury is made digestible, assimilable and acceptable to the tissue cells, it is necessary to make this metal free from these *doṣas* or defects which are either physiological or therapeutic in nature. These *doṣas* or defects are classified in ayurvedic texts into two categories, viz. (1) *naisargika* or defects which are acquired by mercury naturally right at the source, and (2) *anupādhika* (also known as *sapta kañcuka*) which are acquired or introduced into mercury during the process of collection, preservation, storage and distribution. All *doṣas* or defects, if not removed prior to its administration, may cause serious diseases.

Ayurvedic texts are replete with references to these defects or *doṣas* and their adverse effects on the human body. The classification and enumeration, however, are different in different ayurvedic texts composed during different periods of history. It is likely that mercury collected from different mines is possessed with different types of natural and acquired *doṣas* which behave differently when administered to an individual. All these texts are, however, unanimous on the necessity for removing or correcting these defects before the mercury could be used for therapeutic purposes.

Naisargika Doṣas

These *doṣas* or defects are as follows :

1. *Nāga*

In the mine itself, *nāga* or lead gets mixed up with mercury which gives rise to this defect. If not corrected, mercury associated with this *doṣa* may cause ulcers all over the body.

2. *Vaṅga*

In the mine of mercury, *vaṅga* or tin may get mixed up with this metal, and this, if used without rectification may cause obstinate skin diseases including leprosy.

3. *Mala*

Different other types of metallic waste products may get mixed up with mercury and if not corrected, these may cause serious disturbances in the process of digestion and metabolism.

4. *Vahni*

This is caused by the excess of *tejas mahābhūta* in the composition of mercury, and if not corrected its administration may cause serious type of burning sensation all over the body.

5. *Cāpalya*

Pure mercury is by nature very fickle. This fickleness is found in excess in mercury because of the specific nature of the *mahābhautika* composition of this metal. If this defect is not corrected before administration, then it may cause destruction of the sperm and ovum of the males and the females respectively resulting in their impotency, frigidity and even sterility.

6. *Viṣa*

In the mine, it is likely that the mercury is contaminated with many poisonous materials like arsenic. If this defect is not corrected before administration, then it may lead to the death of the patient.

7. *Giri*

Different types of mountains *(giri)* have different types of rocks having different *mahābhautika* composition. That, at times, affects the attributes of mercury. If administered without correcting this defect or *doṣa*, mercury may cause postules all over the body.

8. *Asahyāgni*

Mercury has a fixed boiling point i.e. 357.25° centigrade. But because of certain change in the *mahābhautika* composition of this metal, it may start vapourising even before the stipulated temperature is reached. If mercury associated with this *doṣa* or defect is used in medicine then this may result in unconsciousness of the patient.

Aupādhika or Sapta Kañcuka Doṣas

These are, for the most part physical defects which are acquired by mercury during collection, preservation, storage and distribution. These are formed in the form of layers in the surface of mercury when it comes into contact with oxygen. Physically and chemically pure mercury should not have any reaction when exposed to oxygen in the air. They are called *kañcuka doṣas* because they appear in the surface of the mercury in the form of layers. These are as follows :

1. *Parpaṭī*

If not corrected before administration, it may cause dryness and obstruction to the natural excretion of urine, stool, etc.

2. *Pāṭinī*

If mercury associated with this *doṣa* or defect is administered to a patient, it may cause cracks over the skin of patient.

3. *Bhedī*

If not corrected, this *doṣa* may cause serious type of diarrhoea.

4. *Drāvī*

If mercury associated with this *doṣa* or defect is administered to a patient, it may cause liquification of the tissue elements of the body and retention of more water inside body tissues.

5. *Malakārī*

If mercury associated with this defect is administered, then it will cause aggravation of *vāyu, pitta* and *kapha* (taken together these are called *tri-doṣa*).

6. *Andhakārī*

This *doṣa* or defect may cause blindness of the patient.

7. *Dhvāṅkṣī*

If mercury associated with this *doṣa* or defect is taken without correction or rectification, then it may cause hoarseness of voice.

These defects are described differently in different ayurvedic texts. Some ayurvedic texts have described additional *doṣas* of mercury along with their toxic effects on the human body. However, all of them are unanimous that these defects—both natural and acquired should be corrected before the metal is administered to a patient. A close analysis of the above *doṣas* or defects cannot, however, be made either physically or chemically. They are attributed to the defects in the *mahābhautika* composition of the metal which, of course at a subtler level, are physico-chemical in nature.

Purpose of Śodhana

The literal meaning of the term '*śodhana*' is purification. It is necessary to explain the exact implications of this term. Otherwise, there is a possibility that it will be misinterpreted to mean making mercury and other metals only physically and chemically pure. The term used particularly for *śodhana* or processing of mercury is *saṃskāra*. *Caraka* has explained this term as *guṇāntarādhāna*. By implication, during the process of *saṃskāra* or *śodhana*, the metal or mineral acquires a different property which is useful therapeutically and which overcomes original harmful effects of the metal. To sum up : *śodhana* or *saṃskāra* has following objectives in view :

1. *To make the Metal Suitable for Māraṇa*

The term '*māraṇa*' literally means 'killing'. Metals used as such are heterogeneous to the body tissues, and, therefore, it will not be possible for them to get assimilated into the cells of the tissues to exercise their prescribed therapeutic effects. It will, therefore, be necessary to reduce these metals and minerals including mercury to a fine state of division with such changes in its *mahābhautika* composition as would be homologous with the *mahābhautika* composition of the cells on which the metal has to act to produce the therapeutic effect. This fine state of division of the metal is attained by exposing to the heat of the fire and by repeated trituration or pulverisation. Before exposing the metal to this process, it is necessary to make the component particles fragile and dissociable by reducing their cohesive nature. This is exactly one of the objects of the process of *śodhana* or *saṃskāra*.

2. *To Remove Physical and Chemical Impurities*

In nature, a metal is seldom available in its physically and chemically pure form. The contamination is often natural and it takes place in the mine itself. Some of these metals are available in combination with other metals in the mine in the form of metallic ores or compounds. It is first of all necessary to separate the extraneous objects from the metal. These extraneous objects are, at times, added artificially during commercial transactions. Often contamination takes place knowingly or unknowingly during the process of extraction, storage, preservation and distribution. Therefore, all these extraneous materials are to be removed and the metal should be obtained in physically and chemically pure form for obtaining the desired therapeutic effects.

3. *To Make the Metal Free From Toxicity*

Metals even in their physically and chemically pure form might produce adverse effects because these are inorganic in nature and because of their heterogeneous nature for the tissue cells. By impregnating and triturating with organic material like the juice, decoction etc., of herbs, they are made homologous to the tissue cells, and thus their toxicity is reduced and acceptability to the cells is increased. During this process, certain organic or inorganic materials are actually added to the metal which according to modern science may be explained as addition of impurities.

4. *Transformation of Attributes*

Human body is composed of five *mahābhūtas*, viz. *ākāśa, vāyu, tejas, jala* and *pṛthvī*. In metals and minerals, the fifth, i.e., the *pṛthvī mahābhūta* is predominant. In some of these metals like gold, *tejas mahābūta* is also predominant. Unless the first four *mahābhūtas*, viz., *ākāśa, vāyu, tejas* and *jala* are made potent, it is not likely that these metals and minerals will be able to act effectively as therapeutic agents. *Saṃskāra* or *śodhana* helps in the transformation of these attributes of metals.

5. *Regulation of Physico-Chemical Attributes*

For *deha siddhi* and *lauha siddhi*, it is necessary that the physico-chemical attributes of mercury should be regulated. Mercury is a liquid metal but it is necessary to convert it into a solid form without adding any metal or without making an amalgam of this metal along with other metals. It is necessary that the mercury should be capable of withstanding high temperature and should not be evaporated at about 357° centigrade temperature. It is also necessary that the mercury should be able to digest gold and assimilate it. By implication when gold is added to mercury, the weight of the latter should not increase. This is something which a physicist will think perhaps impossible on the basis of physical laws. But this is exactly the test of mercury (which will be discussed later) before it is taken out for subsequent processing.

All the above mentioned changes are to be made during the process of *śodhana* or *saṃskāra*.

SAṂSKĀRAS OF MERCURY

As has been mentioned before, eighteen different types of *saṃskāras* have been described in ayurvedic texts. Out of these, the first eight *saṃskāras* are essential even if the mercury is to be made suitable for use in ordinary recipes. For *deha siddhi* and *lauha siddhi*, the remaining ten *saṃskāras* are to be performed. If the mercury is to be used for ordinary recipes after the initial eight *saṃskāras*, then it has to be processed further which is called *anuvāsana*. This *kriyā* (type of processing) is, however, not necessary if mercury is to be taken for the remaining ten *saṃskāras*. Therefore, *anuvāsana saṃskāra* is considered as a part of the 8th *saṃskāra* notwithstanding the fact that some physicians take this into account and put the total number of *saṃskāras* to 19. These *saṃskāras* are (1) *svedana*, (2) *mardana*, (3) *mūrcchana*, (4) *utthāpana*, (5) *pātana*, (6) *rodhana* or *bodhana* (*nirodhana* according to *Rasa ratnākara*), (7) *niyāmana*, (8) *dīpana* (or *sandīpana*), (9) *anuvāsana*, (10) *grāsa māna*, (11) *cāraṇa*, (12) *garbha druti*, (13) *bāhya druti*, (14) *jāraṇa*, (15) *rañjana*, (16) *sāraṇa*, (17) *krāmaṇa*, (18) *vedha*, and (19) *śarīra yoga*.

Quantity of Mercury to be Taken for Saṃskāras

Since mercury is a heavy metal and since during the process of *saṃskāras* a portion of this metal gets lost, it should be taken in the beginning in adequate quantity. It is therefore, prescribed that the appropriate quantity for this purpose should be 80 Kg. at a time. However, depending upon the requirement, smaller quantity of mercury can be taken. It can be 1 Kg. or even half a Kg. but in any case it should not be less than 20 Grams.

Auspicious Time

Saṃskāras of mercury should be started on an auspicious time having auspicious constellation. Before starting the work, it is necessary to offer prayer to one's own teacher and Lord Śiva.

Accesories Needed for Śodhana

For different stages of *śodhana,* different types of equipments and implements are needed in addition to herbs, metals and their *sattvas.* However, for the first eight *saṃskāras,* the following equipments are needed : (1) *Pātana yantra,* (2) *Dolā yantra,* (3) *Tapta khalva,* (4) Earthen jar, (5) Enamel trays and bowls, (6) Fine and strong pieces of cloth, (7) *Kāñjī* (a type of vinegar), and (8) Hot water.

Preparation of Kāñjī or Special Type of Vinegar

Different types of corns and cereals as per their availability should be collected and dehusked. These are to be kept inside an earthen jar along with water till the water becomes sour in taste. Into this, drugs like *muṇḍī* (*Sphaeranthus indicus* Linn.), *viṣṇukrāntā* (*Evolvulus alsinoides* Linn.), *punarnavā* (*Boerhaavia diffusa* Linn.), *mīnākṣī* (*Bacopa monnieri* Pennell.), *sahadevī* (*Vernonia cinerea* Less.), *śatāvarī* (*Asparagus racemosus* Willd.), *harītakī* (*Terminalia chebula* Retz.), *bibhītaka* (*Terminalia belerica* Roxb.), *āmalakī* (*Emblica officinalis* Gaertn.) and *citraka* (*Plumbago zeylanica* Linn.) along with their roots and stems should be added as per their availability and kept inside the jar. This preparation is called *dhānyāmalaka* or *kāñjī* and it should be used for different *saṃskāras* of mercury.

SVEDANA SAṂSKĀRA (FOMENTATION)

This is first of the 18 *saṃskāras* to which mercury is subjected both for *deha siddhi* and *lauha siddhi.* Literally the term *'svedana'* means to 'cause sweating or fomentation'. Different methods for this purpose have been prescribed in different ayurvedic texts. Generally following ingredients are used for this purpose :

1. *āsurī* (*Brassica nigra* Koch.);
2. *paṭu* (rock salt);
3. *śuṇṭhī* (*Zingiber officinale* Roscoe);

4. *marica* (*Piper nigrum* Linn.);
5. *pippalī* (*Piper longum* Linn.);
6. *citraka* (*Plumbago zeylanica* Linn.); and
7. *mūlaka* (*Raphanus sativus* Linn.).

The quantity of mercury that should be taken for the purpose of processing has already been discussed. Each of the above mentioned ingredients has to be taken in the quantity of 1/16th of mercury. These are to be soaked in water and made to coarse paste by trituration. A piece of fine and tough cloth should be made four-fold. A layer of *bhūrja patra* (thin layers of the bark of *Betula utilis* D. Don) or banana-leaf is to be spread over this cloth. The surface of this leaf should be smeared with the above mentioned paste and the minimum thickness of the paste should be 3/4th of an inch. Manually, it should be made to the shape of a conical cup and allowed to dry along with the cloth down below and the leaf in between. When it is dried, slowly mercury should be poured into it and the neck of this cup should be closed by putting the remaining paste of the above mentioned drugs. Then the mouth of the cloth should be tied to an iron rod which is kept over the brim of *dolā yantra* (for detailed description of *dolā yantra* see Appendix II). Care should be taken to see that the bottom of this *poṭṭalī* does not touch the bottom of the container, and it remains hanging about 3" above. The size of the pot to be used for *dolā yantra* should be determined on the basis of the quantity of mercury taken for processing. Then the pot of *dolā yantra* should be filled up to 2/3rd of its capacity by *kāñjī*. It has also to be ensured that the upper level of mercury inside the *poṭṭalī* remains below the level of the *kāñjī*. Thereafter, fire should be employed from an oven below. Generally, cow-dung cake is preferred to be used as fuel because of the constant and penetrating nature of its heat. In case of its non-availability, wood of *khadira* (*Acacia catchu* Wild.), *asana* (*Pterocarpus marsupium* Roxb.) or *śāla* (*Shorea robusta* Gaertn.) may be used as fuel.

After the *kāñjī* starts boiling, its level will come down because of evaporation. Its level should be maintained by adding additional *kāñjī*.

About the duration of this process (fomentation), there are different opinions. Heat should be applied constantly for three days minimum if the mercury is to be used for the purpose of *deha siddhi*. But if *lauha siddhi* is aimed at, then fomentation should be applied to mercury continuously for 21 days.

In *rasa śāstra*, the quantum of heat is classified into three categories, viz. (1) *mṛdu* (mild), (2) *madhya* (moderate), and (3) *tīvra* (strong). For this process of *svedana*, only mild fire should be employed and it should never be the third category, i.e., strong fire. If strong fire is employed, there is the possibility of mercury getting evaporated.

Keeping *bhūrja patra* or banana leaf above the fourfold cloth is essential. Apart from their attributes to help in this chemical process, they prevent the fall of mercury from the paste through the cloth into the bottom of the pot of *dolā yantra.* If during fomentation, mercury penetrates through the layer of paste then it will remain above the layer of leaf placed over the cloth, thus permitting the intended chemical action to continue. If mercury comes down then being in touch with the bottom of the pot which remains quite hot during this process, it is likely to get evaporated.

For *dolā yantra,* three types of pots are mentioned to be used. These are (1) earthen pot; (2) iron pot, and (3) copper pot. Even though all three can be used according to convenience, it is always better to use copper pot if available because of the antitoxic property of copper itself. If large quantity of mercury is to be processed, then earthen pot should never be used because it may break during the process resulting in heavy loss.

Some ayurvedic texts suggest that the paste used in this process should be replaced every day. If the processing is to be completed within three days, perhaps such a replacement of pastes is not necessary. But if it is to be continued for 21 days which is necessary for *lauha siddhi* then the paste should be replaced or reinforced. If it is to be replaced then first of all, all the mercury should be recovered and the process is to be started afresh with the new paste. If it is to be supplemented, then paste can be mixed with *kāñjī* and added to the pot of *dolā yantra* frequently which is required to maintain the level of the liquid.

After the *svedana* or fomentation *saṃskāra* is over, it is necessary to get back the mercury. A part of the mercury remains over the paste and another part of it remains over the leaf which is placed below the paste. Generally mercury does not go beyond it and a portion of it gets mixed up with the paste. It is necessary to collect all the globules of mercury from this mixture by gradually washing the paste in an enamelled tray. For washing, warm *kāñjī* or warm water should be used. The herbal drugs of which the paste is prepared, are lighter and during washing, these will gradually come to the upper level of the water and then should be decanted. It should be ensured that the washing is done very slowly so that mercury globules in minute form do not pass away from the enamelled tray with the current of the water. The process should be repeated several times so as to recover maximum quantity of mercury.

If the *dolā yantra* is not prepared properly, if adequate quantity of leaves is not placed below the paste and if the cloth used for tying the leaves and the paste is not very tight, then a part of mercury will fall down and will remain at the bottom of the pot used in *dolā yantra*. If this happens, then the mercury should be carefully salvaged by washing with warm water or warm *kāñjī* and added to the remaining stock.

Effects of Svedana Saṃskāra

By this *saṃskāra* the *mala* or impurities lose their adhesiveness. Since generally acids and alkalies are used in this process it is also possible that a part of these impurities gets dissolved in the liquids and the mercury becomes relatively free from these impurities.

MARDANA SAṂSKĀRA (HOT TRITURATION)

For this *saṃskāra* following ingredients are used :

1. *guḍa* (jaggery);
2. *saindhava* (rock salt);
3. *gṛha dhūma* (house shoot);
4. *dagdhorṇā* (ash of wool);
5. *rājikā (Brassica nigra* Koch.); and
6. *istikā cūrṇa* (powder of brick).

All the above mentioned ingredients are to be taken, each 1/16th of the quantity of mercury, and a paste is to be prepared out of it. The mortar and pestle used in the processing of mercury are either of iron, stone or copper. The stone mortar is likely to develop cracks when heated over fire for a long time and repeatedly. Therefore, as far as possible it should be avoided in this pharmaceutical process. Mercury forms an amalgam with copper. Therefore, if the mortar and pestle are made of copper then there is a possibility of a portion of mercury sticking to this equipment. It is, therefore, proper to use the mortar and pestle made of iron.

First of all, the mortar is to be kept over an oven having strong foundation and charcoal should be ignited. It should be ensured that all through this process, mild heat is constantly emanating from the oven. The powders of above mentioned ingredients should then be added to the mortar and gradually triturated by adding *kāñjī*. To this, mercury should be added and triturated for three days (during day time only). Some physicians continue this trituration process for three days and nights without any break by employing labour in shifts. Some others, however, do this trituration process for 12 hours during day and stop it at night. As the *kāñjī* gets evaporated because of heat below, more and more of it should be added to this mortar.

For *lauha siddhi,* some physicians prefer to continue this process for 21 days, and after each day's work they wash the paste mixed with mercury by hot water or hot *kāñjī* to collect mercury. This is repeated for 21 times. It should be ensured that the trituration is performed slowly so that the mercury does not spill over from the mortar.

After the processing is over, the mercury should be washed with hot water or hot *kāñjī* as was done after the *svedana saṃskāra.* The herbs which are added to the paste will gradually get washed off. It should be ensured that the mercury globules do not go out along with the strong current of water. The process should be done gradually and slowly. Since brick powder is added in the process it is likely to remain along with mercury because of the heaviness of its particles. Therefore, after washing, mercury should be strained through the help of a tough but porous cloth.

According to some alchemical texts, *abhraka sattva* or gold should be added to mercury while trituration and this imparts yellowish tinge to the mercury after this process. This, however, is not necessary at the present stage. If mercury is to be used for *deha siddhi,* addition of *abhraka sattva* or gold is necessary only after eight *saṃskāras*. This will be discussed later.

Effects of Mardana Saṃskāra

By this process, mercury becomes free from *bahirmala* (external excreta) and it also becomes suitable for undergoing subsequent *saṃskāras.*

MŪRCHANA SAṂSKĀRA (FAINTING)

The term *mūrchā* or *mūrchana* means 'fainting'. By this process the mercury loses its natural physico-chemical properties.

For this *saṃskāra* following ingredients are used :

1. *harītakī* (*Terminalia chebula* Retz.);
2. *bibhītakī* (*Terminalia belerica* Roxb.);
3. *āmalakī* (*Emblica officinalis* Gaertn.);
4. *citraka* (*Plumbago zeylanica* Linn.); and
5. *ghṛta kumārī* (*Aloe barbadensis* Mill.).

Each of the above mentioned five ingredients should be 1/16th in weight of mercury. Drugs at No. 1 to No. 4 should be made to a powder and placed in the heated mortar and pestle. To this, juice of *kumārī* should be added and triturated till a paste is formed. Thereafter, mercury should be added and gradually triturated. For heating, the *khalva* should be placed over a strongly based oven and heat should be gradually and continuously applied. Trituration should be continued till mercury loses its cohesiveness and breaks into small globules. It may take more than 3 days for obtaining the state of mercury. To expedite the process, some physicians add the powder of the root of *aṅkola* (*Alangium salviifolium* Wang.). In some books, it is stated that this process should be repeated for seven times but that is necessary for *lauha siddhi*. In some books *tapta khalva* is not directly mentioned to be used but in that case iron mortar and pestle should be used. According to this process, it may take a much longer time to achieve the *mūrchana* stage of mercury.

According to another book, along with all these drugs, mercury should be triturated for one day only. Therefore, it should be collected by washing the paste and then kept inside a crucible *(mūṣā)*. This crucible should then be sealed and cooked in *Bhūdhara yantra* (for description, see App. II) by employing *kukkuṭa* or *kapota puṭa* (for description, see App. II). This process is to be repeated for twenty-one times. But this process is relevant for *lauha siddhi* and not very essential for *deha siddhi*.

Recovery

Since mercury loses its cohesiveness and does not come back to its original shape, it should be recovered very carefully by washing with *kāñjī*, and thereafter, straining through a tough but porous cloth. But the best way to recover mercury after *mūrchana saṃskāra* is to perform *pātana saṃskāra* which is the fourth in the series and it will be discussed hereafter.

Effects of Murchana Saṃskāra

Mardana saṃskāra helps mercury to be free from external excreta but this *mūrchana saṃskāra* makes it free from *naisargika doṣas* i.e., natural poisoning effects inherent in this metal.

UTTHĀPANA SAṂSKĀRA (REVIVAL OF THE NATURAL PHYSICO-CHEMICAL PROPERTIES)

By the previous *(mūrchana) saṃskāra* mercury loses its cohesiveness and it remains in the form of globules. This was necessary to be performed because only by this the inherent toxicity of mercury could be rectified. But unless mercury regains its own physical characteristics, further processing both for *deha siddhi* and *lauha siddhi* will not be possible. It is, therefore, necessary that the original physico-chemical properties of mercury should be restored. This *saṃskāra* is performed by the process of (1) *svedana* (fomentation), (2) *prakṣālana* (repeated washing), (3) *mardana* (trituration), (4) *ātapa* (exposure to sun) and (5) *pātana* (sublimation, distillation, etc.).

Svedana (fomentation) is performed with the help of *dolā yantra.* In the previous *saṃskāra,* mercury was reduced to a globular state and it is often mixed up with the paste. By the application of heat through a *dolā yantra* mercury gradually comes out of the paste and gets accumulated together. Inside the *dolā yantra, kāñjī* should be kept and the mercury which is mixed with the paste of the earlier *saṃskāra* should be kept over banana or banyan leaves well tied through a piece of cloth as described in the first *saṃskāra.* This should be cooked for one day.

Then mercury should be repeatedly washed with the help of warm water or warm *kāñjī* by placing the mercury, mixed with the paste, in an enamelled tray. Because of the heaviness of mercury it will gradually settle down and the paste will come up which should be taken out of the enamelled tray. This, however, should be performed carefully and slowly so that mercury globules do not come out of the enamelled tray along with the strong current of water.

It is likely that mercury will not come to its normal physico-chemical state even by this process and a part of the paste will be still with the mercury. It will, therefore, be necessary to triturate mercury in an iron mortar and pestle which are heated from below (*tapta khalva*). During trituration, small quantities of *kāñjī* should be gradually added to the mortar. Thus, the remaining paste will get easily separated. After this, it will be necessary to pour some more *kāñjī* to make mercury completely free from the paste.

Thereafter, mercury should be exposed to sun and the water inside it should be dried up.

Finally, mercury should be placed in a *Vidyādhara yantra* (for details see App. II). The mercury, because of the heat below will evaporate and get adhered to the bottom of the earthen plate or pot placed at the top. This should be performed for one day and the mercury should, thereafter, be collected.

Some physicians do not consider *utthāpana* as a special type of *saṃskāra*. They consider this as a part of *mūrchana saṃskāra* which helps in the recovery of mercury from the paste. This type of processing for recovery of mercury, according to them, is a must after every *saṃskāra*. But the specific point for discussion here is that unlike *mūrchana saṃskāra*, in other *saṃskāra*, mercury does not lose its physico-chemical properties and it could be recovered in its normal form easily. It is *mūrcchana saṃskāra* which makes mercury to get modified of its physico-chemical properties, and gets thoroughly mixed up with the paste. Therefore, its recovery poses a big problem. Apart from its recovery, it is necessary that the original physico-chemical properties of mercury should be restored, with a view to facilitating other *saṃskāra*. These need elaborate processing because of which *utthāpana* is treated as a special *saṃskāra* and not as a part of *mūrchana saṃskāra*.

PĀTANA SAṂSKĀRA (SUBLIMATION, DISTILLATION, ETC.)

Some ayurvedic texts mention about only one type of *pātana saṃskāra* to be performed. This mostly involves the *tiryak pātana* (distillation). But most of the ayurvedic texts describe three types of *pātana*, viz. *ūrdhva pātana*, *adhaḥ pātana* and *tiryak pātana* to be performed during this *saṃskāra*. In fact, both for *deha siddhi* and *lauha siddhi*, all the three varieties of this *saṃskāra* should be performed.

1. Ūrdhva Pātana (Sublimation)

Mercury which is recovered from *utthāpana saṃskāra* should be triturated in mortar and pestle by adding small pieces of copper, 1/4th in quantity of mercury. To this, the paste of *aṅkola* (*Alangium salviifolium* Wang.), *deva dāru* (*Cedrus deodara* Loud.), *pāṭhā* (*Cissampelos pareira* Linn.), *brāhmī* (*Bacopa monnieri* Pennell.), *citraka* (*Plumbago zeylanica* Linn.), *cāṅgerī* (*Oxalis corniculata* Linn.), *kāka mācī* (*Solanum nigrum* Linn.), *maṇḍūkī* (*Centella asiatica* Urban.), *gaṇikārikā* (*Clerodendrum phlomidis* Linn. f.), *kumārī* (*Aloe barbadensis* Mill.), *jayā* (*Sesbania sesban* Merr.), *bhṛṅga rāja* (*Eclipta alba* Hassk.), *gojihvā* (*Onosma bracteatum* Wall.), *śaṅkha puṣpī* (*Evolvulus alsinoides* Linn.), *pāṭalī* (*Stereospermum suaveolens* DC.), *nirguṇḍī* (*Vitex negundo* Linn.), *kāka jaṅghā (Peristrophe bicalyculata* Nees.), *śatāvarī* (*Asparagus racemosus* Willd.), *ārdraka* (*Zingiber officinale* Rosc.), *deva dālī* (*Luffa echinata* Roxb.), *tila parṇī* (*Gynandropsis pentaphylla* DC.) *nīlikā* (*Indigofera tinctoria* Linn.), *āragvadha* (*Cassia fistula* Linn.) and *kṣīra kanda* (*Ipomoea paniculata* R. Br.) should be added and triturated, for one day. This trituration should take place in a *tapta khalva* (hot mortar and pestle) made of iron. Each of these drugs should be taken in the quantity of 1/16th of mercury. If any of these drugs is not easily available then it can be omitted (and another drug of this group may be used double in quantity) and the *saṃskāra* should be carried out with the help of the remaining drugs. Of course, care should be taken to see that the paste is of adequate quantity.

This mixture of mercury, copper and paste of drugs should be placed at the bottom of *Vidyādhara yantra.* It consists of a big earthen pot, the size of which will vary depending upon the quantity of mercury to be processed. The paste is to be smeared at the inside bottom of this earthen pot. The mouth of the jar will then be covered with the help of an earthen plate. It should be ensured that the size and shape of the plate exactly fit into the mouth of the earthen pot, and the brims of both, viz., the lower earthern pot and the upper earthen plate should be sealed with the help of seven layers of mud-smeared cloth. Then it should be dried in sun. The convex side of the earthen plate should remain inside the pot and the concave side should be above. Then this *yantra* should be placed over fire, and in the plate kept above, cold water should be kept. Because of the heat below, the water will gradually become warm and this should be immediately taken out and replaced by cold water. This should be done repeatedly so that the bottom of the earthen plate remains always cold. The process is to be continued for about twelve hours and then the fire should be discontinued.

Next day when the pot is cooled down, the seal should be gradually and slowly broken, and mercury adhered to the bottom of the earthen plate should be slowly scrapped into an enamel tray with the help of a knife. While breaking the seal, the pot should be handled very gently so that the sublimed mercury does not fall down and get mixed up with the paste at the bottom of the earthen jar. The mercury, thus, collected in the enamel tray should be washed with the help of warm water or warm *kāñjī* and collected for subsequent processing. For *deha siddhi, ūrdhva pātana* only once is enough but for *lauha siddhi* it has to be performed for seven times.

This makes mercury free from some of the residual *doṣas* or defects.

2. *Adhaḥ Pātana*

For *adhaḥ pātana*, either *Vidyādhara yantra* or *Ḍamaru yantra* should be used. In *Ḍamaru yantra*, instead of the upper plate, a second earthen jar is taken. It should be ensured that the brims of both the earthen jars fit to each other. Mercury should be triturated with the paste of *harītakī* (*Terminalia chebula* Retz.), *bibhītakī* (*Terminalia belerica* Roxb.), *āmalakī* (*Emblica officinalis* Gaertn.), *rājikā* (*Brassica nigra* Koch.), *śigru* (*Moringa oleifera* Lam.), *śuṇṭhī* (*Zingiber officinalis* Rosc.), *pippalī* (*Piper longum* Linn.), *marica* (*Piper nigrum* Linn.), *lavaṇa* (rock salt) and *citraka* (*Plumbago zeylanica* Linn.). All these drugs should be taken in quantity equal to that of mercury individually. It should be triturated with the help of *kāñjī* for one day. This paste should be smeared over the inside bottom of the upper jar and then dried. The upper jar should then be kept inverted over the lower jar and the brims of both the jars should be sealed with seven layers of mud smeared cloth and dried. Then a pit should be dug in the earth. The size of the pit should be such that the lower jar could be easily kept inside it. Over the upper jar heat should be employed, and for this purpose *laghu puṭa* (for details see App. II) should be employed. The lower jar should be kept cool by frequently adding water to the earth around it. Some physicians prefer to give heat with the help of twenty cow-dung cakes. The process of heating should be allowed to continue till the fire of the cow-dung cake is extinguished. After it becomes cool, the *Ḍamaru yantra* should be taken out of the earth and the seal should be carefully broken. From the lower jar mercury should be collected.

3. *Tiryak Pātana*

This is an important step for the processing of mercury particularly during the fifth *saṃskāra* because some physicians prefer to perform this *tiryak pātana* three times instead of once each of *ūrdhva pātana, adhaḥ pātana* and *tiryak pātana*. For the process of *tiryak pātana*, mercury should be mixed with *dhānyābhraka* (for details, see the chapter dealing with *abhra* or mica), *harītakī* (*Terminalia chebula* Retz.), *bibhītakī* (*Terminalia belerica* Roxb.), *āmalakī* (*Emblica officinalis* Gaertn.), *rājikā* (*Brassica nigra* Koch.), *śigru* (*Moringa oleifera* Lam.), *śuṇṭhī* (*Zingiber officinale* Rosc.), *pippalī* (*Piper longum* Linn.), *marica* (*Piper nigrum* Linn.), *lavaṇa* (rock salt) and *citraka* (*Plumbago zeylanica* Linn.)--each taken in equal quantity and the quantity of all these drugs should be same as that of mercury. It should be triturated by adding small quantity of *kāñjī* till mercury loses its own physical form. Then this paste should be kept inside the *Tiryak pātana yantra* (for details, see Appendix II). *Tiryak pātana yantra* in ancient times was prepared with the help of earthen vessels but for sake of convenience it is now a days prepared of iron. It consists of a cylindrical iron jar with a narrow mouth to which a bent iron pipe is screwed. The other end of the iron pipe is placed inside a vessel containing water. For sake of convenience, the outer end of this iron pipe is connected with a rubber pipe which opens into a glass jar. This glass jar is kept inside a container having cold water. The cylindrical iron jar is placed over an oven and heat is employed. The joints of the mouth of the cylindrical jar and the iron pipe are sealed with the help of seven layers of mud-smeared cloth and dried beforehand. When the heat is employed to the iron jar containing the mercury and the paste of the drugs, the mercury will evaporate and through the bent iron pipe pass into the glass bottle kept inside the water pot. The bent iron pipe should be wrapped with cloth and cold water should be poured over it to keep it cool. This process can also be performed by any glass distilling apparatus, provided the glass is strong and thermostable.

To the iron jar containing mercury and paste of drugs, strong heat should be applied from an oven and it should be continued till all the mercury comes out of the paste.

Earth for Sealing Joints

Mercury evaporates in 357° centigrade of heat and if the joints of these equipments are not properly sealed then it may result in the leaking of mercury resulting in considerable loss. Therefore, it should be ensured that the seal is made properly and the earth used for sealing is of appropriate type. It should be resistant to both fire and water. For this purpose two types of clay are described in ayurveda, viz., *vahni mṛtsnā* (fire clay) and *jala mṛtsnā* (water clay). Fire clay or *vahni mṛtsnā* is prepared by the powder of chalk (talcum), salt and *maṇḍūra* (iron rust). All the three taken in equal quantities should be well triturated by adding buffalo-milk. This clay is heat resistant, i.e., it does not get broken or burnt even if it comes in direct contact with fire. *Jala mṛtsnā* (water clay), on the other hand, is prepared by the decoction of the bark of *babūla* (*Acacia arabica* Willd.). This decoction should be further boiled so that it becomes thicker. To this, the fine powder of *maṇḍūra* (iron rust) and the powder of jaggery in equal quantities should be added and triturated. If the seal made out of this clay is applied and dried, then water even if it is boiling, will not be able to break it. Appropriately both types of clay should be used in the above mentioned *pātana yantra*.

BODHANA OR RODHANA SAṂSKĀRA (REVIVAL OF POTENCY)

This sixth *saṃskāra* is also called *śodhana*. Because of the previous five *saṃskāras*, the mercury becomes absolutely free from toxicity (*doṣa*). This is an important achievement because ultimately for *deha siddhi* it is to be administered to human beings and there should not be any adverse effect. But these *saṃskāras* (1st to 5th) bring about such molecular chage in this metal by which it loses some of its physico-chemical properties inasmuch as its therapeutic potency becomes very mild. Not only for *deha siddhi* but also for *lauha siddhi* it becomes ineffective because its power to get mixed up with other metals (which will be described in detail later), to digest them and to assimilate them becomes mild.

Therefore, both for *deha siddhi* and *lauha siddhi*, its original potency should be restored, and this is the purpose of this *rodhana saṃskāra*. The simplest way to reviving is to keep mercury in an earthen jar and to this a solution of rock-salt *(saindhava)* should be added. The jar should then be covered, sealed and kept inside a pit dug in the earth. This will revive the potency of mercury for the purpose of *deha siddhi*. But for *lauha siddhi*, it is necessary that this mercury should be kept inside a cup made of *bhūrja patra* (thin layers of the bark of *Betula utilis* D. Don) and this should be tied up in a piece of cloth. In a *dolā yantra* this mercury should be boiled by adding cow's urine or lemon juice.

For the preparation of solution of rock-salt, it is necessary to mix salt with five times of water.

Thereafter, mercury should be placed in an enamel tray and washed with warm *kāñjī* or warm water.

NIYĀMANA SAṂSKĀRA (REGULATION OF PHYSICAL PROPERTIES)

By *rodhana saṃskāra* mercury regains its lost potency. But for future processing it is necessary that its fickleness should be regulated. The paste of *tāmbūla* (*Piper betle* Linn.), *laśuna* (*Allium sativum* Linn.), *saindhava* (rock-salt), *bhṛṅga rāja* (*Eclipta alba* Hassk.), *vandhyā karkoṭī* (*Luffa cylindrica* M. Roem.) and *ciñcā* (*Tamarindus indica* Linn.), each taken 1/16th in quantity of mercury, should be spread over the leaves of banana or banyan which are spread over a thick piece of cloth. Then the cloth should be tied with the help of a string and the whole thing should be cooked in *Dolā yantra* by adding *kāñjī*. Thereafter, mercury should be recovered from the paste by washing with the help of warm water or warm *kāñjī* in an enamel tray. This process reduces the fickleness of mercury.

In addition to the arrests of fickleness it is also necessary to make mercury thermostable. For this purpose, a crucible should be prepared of a piece of rock-salt. Inside this crucible, mercury, *navasāda* (Ammonium chloride) and lemon juice should be added. Thereafter, the mouth of crucible should be sealed. It should then be kept inside a pit and covered with 5" of earth. Then fire should be applied with the help of cow-dung cakes for twenty one days. It is likely that the crucible of rock-salt might not stand the heat for 21 days at a stretch. It will, therefore, be necessary to replace the crucible with a new one every subsequent days. At the next stage of this process, mercury should be kept inside a glass jar by adding the powder of rock-salt and sealed. This glass jar should be kept inside a pit dug in the earth for twenty-one days. Application of heat during this stage is not necessary. By exposing mercury to these all stages of processing, which takes about forty-two days, it becomes resistant to the action of fire i.e. its evaporation point becomes more than 357° centigrade.

Thus by this *niyāmana saṃskāra*, mercury becomes full of lustre. It losses its fickleness. It becomes more stable and its evaporation point is increased.

DĪPANA SAṂSKĀRA

In a *dolā yantra* mercury should be kept over the paste of *saurāṣṭrī* (alum), *kāsīsa* (Iron sulphate), *ṭaṅkaṇa* (borax), *śigru* (*Moringa oleifera* Lam.), *marica* (*Piper nigrum* Linn.), *sainddhava* (rock-salt) and *rājikā* (*Brassica nigra* Koch), each taken 1/16th in quantity of mercury, and cooked by adding *kāñjī*. This process should be continued for three days continuously.

Thereafter, mercury should be recovered by washing the paste taken out of *dolā yantra* in an enamel tray with the help of warm *kāñjī* or warm water. As before, every care should be taken to wash the paste very slowly so that mercury in small particles does not go out of the enamel tray because of strong current of water or *kāñjī*.

ANUVĀSANA SAṂSKĀRA

As has been mentioned earlier, *anuvāsana* for all practical purposes is not treated as a separate *saṃskāra*. However, this helps in increasing the potency of mercury. In this *saṃskāra*, mercury is mixed with lime juice, *śuṇṭhī* (*Zingiber officinale* Rosc.), *saindhava* (rock-salt), *citraka* (*Plumbago zeylanica* Linn.) and *hiṅgu* (asafoetida), each taken 1/16th in quantity of mercury. This should be exposed to sun for 21 days. Thereafter, by washing with warm water or warm *kāñjī*, mercury may be recovered.

Eight Saṃskāras

Excluding *anuvāsana*, the remaining eight *saṃskāras* are essential for both *deha siddhi* and *lauha siddhi* and even for the preparation of ordinary medicines. Mercury should not be used for internal medication without these eight *saṃskāras*. There are several methods prescribed in ayurvedic texts which are simple, less time consuming and inexpensive to make mercury free from toxicity. But the main purpose of using mercury in medicine is to get its therapeutic potency for promotion of positive health and prevention as well as cure of diseases. This could, however, be achieved only if mercury is processed through the eight *saṃskāras* described later, are meant both for *deha siddhi* and *lauha siddhi*. These *saṃskāras* make mercury potent for curing in a short time, some of the obstinate and otherwise incurable diseases, and this metal, added to various recipes, works as a potent rejuvenating agent.

GRĀSA MĀNA SAṂSKĀRA

Grāsa māna, *cāraṇa* (11th *saṃskāra*), *drutis* (12th and 13th *saṃskāras*) and *jāraṇa* (14th *saṃskāra*)--all these four *saṃskāras* are nothing but a single continuous process. In *grāsa māna saṃskāra*, the quantity of metal that should be added to mercury is determined. In *cāraṇa*, the metal in appropriate quantity is mixed with the mercury. In *druti*, the metal gets digested and in *jāraṇa saṃskāra* the metal gets finally assimilated into the mercury without increasing its weight. To illustrate the quantity of food required for an individual is determined by *grāsa māna*. Chewing of food is performed by *cāraṇa*; digestion of food is achieved by *druti* and *jāraṇa* represents assimilation of food by the tissues of the body. Since *grāsa māna* involves only the determination of the quantity of metal to be added to mercury, it is not treated as a separate *saṃskāra* according to some physicians. On the other hand, they take into account *anuvāsana* which is already described as one of the *saṃskāras*. *Grāsa māna*, according to them, forms a part of *cāraṇa saṃskāra*.

Bīja

The metal that is added to mercury at this stage is called *bīja* (lit. seed). For *lauha siddhi* that is intended to prepare gold out of mercury, the *bīja* should be *nāga* or lead. If the purpose is to prepare silver out of mercury, then *vaṅga* or tin should be used as *bīja* or seed. If, however, *deha siddhi* is to be achieved, gold should be used as *bīja.* But for both *deha siddhi* and *lauha siddhi,* in the beginning, *abhraka* (mica) in *bhasma* form should be used as seed or *bīja.* For this purpose black variety of mica which is called *vajrābhraka* (biotite mica) should be used. Some physicians prefer to use the *sattva* (essence) of mica as *bīja* at this stage because it gets easily assimilated into mercury and increases its potency.

Whatever it may be, the *bīja* should be 1/64th of mercury in the beginning. After its *jāraṇa* or assimilation is over, again this *bīja* should be added to mercury in the quantity of 1/32nd part of mercury. This should be followed by *jāraṇa* of 1/16th in quantity of *bīja,* 1/8th in quantity of *bīja* and 1/4th in quantity of *bīja.* To recapitulate : in the beginning the *bhasma* of *abhraka* (biotite mica) or its *sattva* or essence (the process of extracting *sattva* from mica will be described later) should be used as *bīja.* Thereafter, for *deha siddhi* 1/64th, 1/32nd, 1/16th, 1/8th and 1/4th parts (in comparison to the quiantity of mercury) of gold should be used as *bija.* If the purpose is only to achieve *lauha siddhi* i.e., to prepare gold out of mercury then 1/64th, 1/32nd, 1/16th, 1/8th, and 1/4 in parts, (of the quantity of mercury) of lead should be used as *bīja.* If it is intended to prepare silver out of mercury, then 1/64th, 1/32nd, 1/16th, 1/8th and 1/4th parts (of the quantity of mercury) of tin should be used as *bīja.*

This determination of the quantity of *bīja* or seed is called *grāsa māna (grāsa*=food and *māna*=measurement).

CĀRAṆĀ SAṂSKĀRA

As has been mentioned before, *cāraṇa, drutis* (both the types) and *jāraṇa,* these four *saṃskāras* are performed continuously. The main aim of these four *saṃskāras* is to enable mercury to assimilate the metals which are added to it. In the previous *saṃskāra* i.e., *grāsa māna,* different types of metals are to be added and their quantities are already described. As has been described before, *cāraṇa* represents the chewing of food, both types of *druti* represent the process of digestion, and *jāraṇa* represents the process of assimilation.

Before undertaking these *saṃskāras* three factors should be ensured, viz., (1) *pārada* or mercury is free from toxicity, (2) the requisite hunger has been created inside the mercury to assimilate metals, and (3) it should be relatively more stable over fire i.e. it should be able to resist strong heat before getting evaporated.

By the *saṃskāras* described before, mercury has become free from toxicity, its appetite to digest other metals has increased and it has become more heat resistant. But the latter two aspects are not sufficiently developed. Therefore, some more preparatory measures are required to be taken. Mercury should be exposed to *svedana* (fomentation) with the help of *dolā yantra* again for seven times. The process to be followed for *svedana* has already been described and the same procedure has to be adopted at present. But in the place of *kāñjī*, the fomentation should be given with the help of drugs belonging to *kṣāra varga*, *lavaṇa varga* and *amla varga* separately. Drugs belonging to these groups are as follows:

Kṣāra Varga (Group of Alkali Drugs)

These are *tila* (*Sesamum indicum* Linn.), *apāmārga* (*Achyranthes aspera* Linn.), *kadalī* (*Musa paradisiaca* Linn.), *mūlaka* (*Raphanus sativus* Linn.), *palāśa* (*Butea monosperma* Kuntze.), *śobhāñjana* (*Moringa oleifera* Lam.), *citraka* (*Plumbago zeylanica* Linn.) and *ārdraka* (*Zingiber officinale* Rosc.). All these drugs or any of these readily available should be taken for the preparation of *kṣāra* (alkali). These are to be burnt by *antardhūma* method i.e. without free air. These drugs are to be kept inside an earthen jar covered with an earthen plate, the joint is sealed and then the jar is kept over fire for about six hours. By this, the drug gets burnt and reduced to ash. This ash is collected, mixed with adequate quantity of water and strained through a cloth. Thereafter, the whole thing is allowed to settle down. Fine particles of the ash will then settle down at the bottom of the jar and the water will remain above which is slowly decanted. Then for removing the residual water, the jar should be kept over mild fire or it is exposed to sun for getting dried up. Often it is convenient to adopt both of them. Thus at the end, the dry powder containing small particles of alkaline material will be available. Then by adding six times of water, it is to be used in *Dolā yantra* for *svedana* or fomentation.

Lavaṇa Varga (Group of Salts)

These include rock-salt, sea-salt, sonchal-salt and *nausādara* (Aluminium chloride). Saturated solution of all or any of these salts readily available should be prepared and this solution is to be used in *Dolā yantra* for *svedana* or fomentation.

Amla Varga (Group of Sour Drugs)

These include *amla vetasa* (*Garcinia pedunculata* Roxb.), *jambīra* (*Citrus limon* Burm. f.), *bīja pūraka* (*Citrus medica* Linn.), *cāṅgerī* (*Oxalis corniculata* Linn.), *nāraṅga* (*Citrus reticulata* Blanc.) and *tintiḍī* (*Rhus parviflora* Roxb.). Juice of these drugs should be used in *Dolā yantra* for *svedana* or fomentation.

After these three fomentations, mercury becomes capable of digesting the metals to be added and its appetite is sufficiently increased.

For *pakṣa cheda* (to increase the vapourisation point), it is essential that the *bhasma* of *abhraka* (mica) or *abhraka sattva* (essence of mica) should be added to the mercury and processed. Between *abhraka bhasma* and *abhraka sattva* the latter should be used for *lauha siddhi* and the former is enough for *deha siddhi*.

Extraction of Abhraka Sattva

It takes a long time for the *bhasma* of *abhraka* (mica) to get mixed up into mercury and it involves a lot of labour. On the other hand, it is easier for mercury to digest and assimilate *abhraka sattva*. Therefore, both for *deha siddhi* and *lauha siddhi*, it is better to use *abhraka sattva* in this process. If the *sattva* of *mākṣika* (copper pyrite) is added to it, then the process becomes all the more easier. For the preparation of *abhraka sattva*, *vajrābhraka* (biotite mica) should be taken. The powder of mica should be soaked (impregnated) with milk, curd, ghee, cow-dung and cow-urine. All these five taken together are called *pañca gavya*. With these ingredients, mica should be impregnated and triturated for twelve hours. Then the paste should be taken in a crucible and kept over strong fire which is inflamed with the help of a blower for about six hours. By this process the metallic essence of *abhraka* separates inside the crucible. This should be collected and used as such or in a *bhasma* form for *cāraṇa*. The colour of the *sattva* is like that of iron or slightly yellowish. The same process should be followed for the extraction of *sattva* from *mākṣika* (copper pyrite). Some physicians add 10% of borax and 10% of the powder of *samudra phala* (*Barringtonia acutangula* Gaertn.) to mica. This helps in getting the *sattva* quickly and easily.

Two Types of Cāraṇa

Cāraṇa is of two types, viz. *samukha* or *sabīja cāraṇa* and *nirmukha* or *nirbīja cāraṇa*. By *samukha cāraṇa*, the digestive power of mercury is further stimulated. It is an improvement over the *dīpana saṃskāra* (8th step). The first stage of this process is called *mukhī karaṇa*. Usually the *bhasma* of *abhraka* (mica) or *abhraka sattva* is used as *bīja* (seed) in this process. The method of preparing *abhraka sattva* is already described above. For *mukhī karaṇa*, mercury is triturated by adding the paste of earth-worm for three days. The paste should then be kept inside a crucible the inside wall of which is smeared with the paste of earth-worm and the remaining space over the paste of mercury should also be filled with more of the paste of earth-worm. The mouth of the crucible should then be sealed with cow-dung and it should be kept inside a pit dug in the earth. Over this, cow-dung fire should be applied. This process is to be repeated for thirty times.

The *sattva* of *abhraka* (mica) should also be further processed before adding to this mercury. This process is called *abhiṣeka*.

Abhiṣeka of Abhra Sattva

For *abhiṣeka*, the *sattva* of *abhraka* (mica) should be impregnated and triturated for seven days by adding the juice or decoction of rhizome of banana, *mūlaka* (*Raphanus sativus* Linn.), *śatāvarī* (*Asparagus racemosus* Willd.), *punarnavā* (*Boerhaavia diffusa* Linn.), *megha nāda* (*Amaranthus tricolor* Linn.), *yava* (barley), *ciñcā* (*Tamarindus indica* Linn.), *śigru* (*Moringa oleifera* Lam.) and *sūraṇa* (*Amorphophallus companulatus* Blume.).

Purified sulphur should be melted by adding equal quantity of purified *bhasma* of *abhraka*. To this paste, equal quantity of processed mercury should be added and triturated. This should be covered all around with the paste of sulphur and *nāga* or lead (if the intention is to prepare gold) or sulphur and copper (if the intention is to achieve *deha siddhi*). In a *dolā yantra* (see App. II), this should be cooked by adding melted sulphur for three days. This process is called *garbha karma*. Thereafter, mercury should be taken out of this compound by distillation. Again the same process should be repeated for three days. This second process is called *piṣṭa karma*. Then the mercury should be taken out by distillation and the process should be repeated by adding more of *bīja* i.e. *abhraka bhasma* or *abhraka sattva* as described in the *grāsa māna saṃskāra*.

There are several other methods of this *samukha cāraṇa saṃskāra* which are described in different ayurvedic texts on *rasa śāstra*. *Nirmukha* or *nirbīja cāraṇa* is done by triturating mercury with *divya auṣadhis* (see App. I). To sixty-four parts of mercury, four parts of *vaikrānta* (tourmaline) and one part of the *bhasma* of diamond should be added and triturated by adding the juice of plants belonging to the group called *Divya auṣadhis* (see App. I). By this, mercury becomes capable of digesting *bījas* (seeds) as described in *grāsa māna saṃskāra.*

GARBHA DRUTI (INTERNAL DIGESTION)

Druti is of two types, viz., *garbha* (internal) *druti* and *bāhya* (external) *druti. Cāraṇa saṃskāra* represents the chewing of the food. Now it is required to be digested. This can be achieved either by *garbha druti* or by *bāhya druti.* While describing *grāsa māna saṃskāra,* it has been explained that the *bīja* of *abhraka* (mica) or *abhraka sattva* is to be added to mercury in different proportions till *jāraṇa saṃskāra* is achieved. Thereafter, the *bīja* of either *nāga* (lead) or *vaṅga* (tin) is to be added for *lauha siddhi* (*nāga* or lead is to be added if the intention is to prepare gold, and *vaṅga* or tin is to be added if the intention is to prepare silver).

Biḍa

For *druti* of different metals, different types of *biḍa* (catalytic agents) is to be added. There are general types of *biḍa* and there are *biḍas* specific to each metal. The former type is preparped by *sauvarcala* (sonchal salt), *śuṇṭhī* (*Zingber officinale* Rosc.), *pippalī* (*Piper longum* Linn.), *marica* (*Piper nigrum* Linn.), *sphaṭikā* (alum), *kāsīsa* (iron sulphate) and *gandhaka* (sulphur).

All these drugs taken in equal quantities, are to be impregnated with the juice of *śobhāñjana* (*Moringa oleifera* Lam.) for one hundred times. By more impregnation and trituration, the *biḍa* becomes more and more effective. This *biḍa* is added to mercury, 1/8th in quantity. The *biḍa* is to be kept below and above mercury for processing. For the *garbha druti* of gold, special type of *biḍa* is needed. This is prepared by the *kṣāra* (alkali) prepared of *mūlaka* (*Raphanus sativus* Linn.) by adding cow's urine. Gold is to be impregnated and triturated by adding this alkali preparation for one hundred times. This *biḍa* helps in immediate *druti* (digestion) and *jāraṇa* (assimilation) of gold in mercury.

Mercury mixed with the *bīja* (after *cāraṇa saṃskāra*) is to be added with equal quantity of sulphur, and *kajjalī* (fine black powder like collyrium) is to be prepared. To this, *biḍa,* 1/8th in quantity, is to be added. Cow's urine should be added to it and triturated till it becomes a paste. This paste is to be smeared inside a crucible *(mūṣā)* specially prepared for this purpose. In an earthen pot, at the bottom, *haritāla* (orpiment), *manaḥ śilā* (realgar) or *gandhaka* (sulphur) is to be kept in powder form in appropriate quantity. Over it, the crucible smeared with the paste of mercury etc., should be placed inverted i.e. with its face downwards. Then the earthen pot is to be placed over an oven. Cow-dung should be used as fuel in the oven. As the earthen pot gets heated up the fumes of *manaḥ śilā* (realgar), etc. will come up. A part of the fume will also go into the crucible. Very mild heat should be applied till the whole of *manaḥ śilā*, etc. are burnt. It takes about six to twelve hours. This process helps in *garbha druti*.

BĀHYA DRUTI (DIGESTION—EXTERNAL)

In the *garbha druti* described above, different metals which are added as *bīja* get digested while kept inside the mercury. In *bāhya druti* the metal is reduced to liquid form outside and then added to mercury before *jāraṇa*. This process, therefore, is not required if the metal is already added according to *garbha druti* method. If, however, *bāhya druti saṃskāra* is to be performed, then one can avoid both *cāraṇa* and *garbha druti saṃskāras* described above. The quantity of the metal to be added to the mercury should, however, be on the lines suggested in *grāsa māna* and *garbha druti saṃskāras*. For *bāhya druti*, the fruit of *kapi tinduka* (*Feronia limonia* Swingle) is to be made to a powder and it has to be impregnated and triturated with goat's urine for one hundred times. After each time of impregnation and trituration, the paste should be dried by exposing to sun. This powder should be added to the *abhraka* (mica) *bhasma* or *abhraka sattva*, kept in a crucible and heated over fire. After this, the metal should be poured over a pot containing til oil. This process has to be repeated for three times for getting the metal in appropriate liquid form. For *bāhya druti* of gold, the powder of *deva dālī* (*Luffa echinata* Roxb.) should be impregnated with its juice for one hundred times. After each impregnation and trituration it should be dried in shade. First of all, gold should be heated till it melts. To this, the powder of *deva dālī* described above, should be added. By this, gold remains in liquid form. In the same way other metals can be reduced to a liquid form. This liquid metal should be added to mercury, and the powder of *kṛṣṇa aguru* (*Aquilaria agallocha* Roxb.), *kastūrī* (musk), sugar, garlic, white variety of asafoetida, sulphur and the powder of the seed of *palāśa* (*Butea monosperma* Kuntze) should be added. The whole thing should be triturated in a *tapta khalva* (hot mortar and pestle) made of iron. This process is called *dvandva melāpana* (lit. combination of two items).

Some scholars do not follow the rules regarding the quantity of metal to be added to mercury as described in *grāsa māna saṃskāra*. They add mercury to the liquefied metal in equal quantity only. But it is better to add the liquid metal in gradually increased quantities, viz. sixteen times, thirty-two times and even sixty four times of mercury. This makes the mercury progressively more and more potent. Mercury which has digested the liquid metal taken in the quantity of sixty-four times becomes most potent.

JĀRAṆA SAṂSKĀRA (ASSIMILATION)

Garbha druti and *bāhya druti*, both represent the digestion of the metal (which is added in the form of *bīja*) by mercury. The next step is *jāraṇa* or complete assimilation of the metal by mercury. If this *jāraṇa* or assimilation takes place, then the mercury in spite of the addition of other metals will not change in weight. This is the actual test for the successful completion of *jāraṇa saṃskāra*. This *saṃskāra*, as has been mentioned before, starts right from *cāraṇa saṃskāra* and *garbha druti* (including *bāhya druti*). But in *cāraṇa* and *garbha druti* there will be some increase in the weight of mercury because of the weight of the added metal. But at the state of *jāraṇa* there should be no increase in the weight of mercury. For *jāraṇa saṃskāra* along with the *bīja*, *biḍa* (described before) is essential, and the processing is done over *tapta khalva*.

Jāraṇa is of two types, viz., *bāla jāraṇa* and *vṛddha jāraṇa*. *Bāla jāraṇa* is performed with a view to making mercury suitable for curing diseases and also for rejuvenation therapy. It can be performed even after the eighth i.e. *dīpana saṃskāra*. It is generally done by adding sulphur to mercury in different proportions and by cooking in a *Vālukā yantra* (see Appendix II). *Vṛddha jāraṇa* is meant for both *deha siddhi* and *lauha siddhi*.

Khoṭa

This is done with the help of *bījas* and *biḍas* described before. For the purpose of *jāraṇa*, mercury should be added with 1/4th in quantity of sulphur and triturated by adding the juice of *śatāvarī* (*Asparagus racemosus* Willd.), *tāmbūla* (*Piper betle* Linn.), *laśuna* (*Allium sativum* Linn,), *bhṛṅga rāja* (*Eclipta alba* Hassk.), *vandhyā karkoṭakī* (*Momordica cochinchinensis* Spreng.) and the solution of rock-salt. The process should be performed over heated iron mortar and pestle. Because of the addition of *abhraka sattva* in the earlier *saṃskāra*, mercury has already become thermostable. Similarly, sulphur is made themostable by adding *tuttha* (Copper sulphate) and *navasādara* (Ammonium chloride), both taken in quantities equal to that of sulphur.

Thereafter, the paste should be made to small pills of the size of ber fruit and dried in shade. These dried pills should be kept in an iron pan and covered with an iron plate. The joint of the pan and the plate should be properly sealed with seven layers of mud smeared cloth (the mud should be mixed with rock-salt). This iron pan should then be placed over an oven which contains fire of smokeless charcoal. Then with the help of a blower, the fire should be further inflammed to produce strong heat. As a result of this, both the iron pan and the iron plate become red hot. Thereafter, the iron pan should be allowed to cool down of its own. By this process, the mercury and sulphur inside the pan melt and become red in colour. This condition of mercury is called *khoṭa*. Then the seal should be broken, and the mercury and sulphur, mixed together in the shape of a bolus and red in colour should be collected. This red bolus should be kept inside the *vajra mūṣā* (see Appendix II) and heated till it melts. This molten compound should be poured over oil by which it becomes solid again.

To this, 1/4th of *ṭaṅkaṇa* (borax) and equal quantity of *vaṅga* (tin) should be added. This should be kept over the oven by which it melts. This process should be repeated three times as a result of which three times of *vaṅga* (tin) will have to be added to this compound. To this, a small quantity (5%) of *nāga* (lead) should be added. This compound will be useful for *lauha siddhi* and it is not useful for *deha siddhi*. If it is intended to be used for *deha siddhi* then *nāga* (lead) should not be added. It should be ensured that for *deha siddhi* all metals to be added during these processes should have undergone the process of *śodhana* (purification).

RAÑJANA SAṂSKĀRA (COLOURATION)

The term *rañjana* means 'colouration'. The compound of mercury collected from the previous *saṃskāra* should be used for *rañjana saṃskāra*. For this purpose, the *bīja* should first of all be exposed to *rañjana saṃskāra*. Apart from the general method, for different types of *bījas* different methods have been prescribed. The general method includes the preparation of *Rañjana taila*.

Rañjana Taila

The flower of *palāśa* (*Butea monosperma* Kuntze), *mañjiṣṭhā* (*Rubia cordifolia* Linn.), red variety of *karavīra* (*Nerium indicum* Mill.), *khadira* (*Acacia catechu* Willd.), *rakta candana* (*Pterocarpus santalinus*

Linn. f.), *niśā (Curcuma longa* Linn.), *dāru niśā* (*Berberis aristata* DC.), *sarala* (*Pinus roxburghii* Sarg.), *deva dāru* (*Cedrus deodara* Loud.) and *japā* (*Hibiscus rosa-sinensis* Linn.) should be made to a paste by adding the decoction of *lākṣā* (lac). To this, four times of sesame oil should be added. This should be added further, with the decoction and juice of the above mentioned drugs, four times in quantity in total. The oil should be cooked according to the prescribed method.

The *bīja* which is to be used for *rañjana saṃskāra* is first to be heated and immersed in this oil (*Rañjana taila*). This should be done at least for twenty one times by which red colour is imparted to the *bīja*. The *bīja* of *nāga* or lead is used if it is proposed to prepare gold out of mercury in *dhātu siddhi*. For *deha siddhi*, the *bīja* of gold is generally used and processed according to the above mentioned procedure.

For *dhātu vāda*, a special method of *rañjana saṃskāra* is generally followed. In an iron pan, the *bīja* i.e. *nāga* or lead is to be kept and heated over an oven till lead starts melting. During this process of melting, the powder of leaves and seeds of *palāśa* (*Butea monosperma* Kuntze) should be added in small quantities and triturated with the help of a stick made of the wood of *palāśa* (*Butea monosperma* Kuntze). In about twelve hours, the lead will be reduced to *bhasma* form. To this, equal quantity of sulphur should be added and triturated by adding lemon juice for three hours. This should then be kept inside two earthen plates the border of which is sealed properly and cooked by *gaja puṭa* (see App. II). After it is cooled down, the compound should be removed and again added with 1/4th in quantity of sulphur. This should then be kept in earthen plates as before and again cooked in *gaja puṭa*. This process should be repeated for fourteen times. This imparts red colour to *nāga* (lead).

A powder should be made of all the five parts of *vāsā* (*Adhatoda vasica* Nees.), bark of *kakubha* (*Terminalia arjuna* W. & A.), flower of *śigru* (*Moringa oleifera* Lam.), *Palāśa* (*Butea monosperma* Kuntze), *śāka* (*Tectona grandis* Linn. f.), *nāga vallī* (*Piper betle* Linn.), *ahimāra* (*Acacia leucophloea* Willd.) and *kumārī* (*Aloe barbadensis* Mill.). To this, two parts of *manaḥ śilā* (realgar) should be added and boiled by adding four times of cow's urine till 1/4th remains. To this liquid, the above mentioned *bhasma* of *nāga* (lead) should be added and cooked over an oven for seven days. During cooking, it should be stirred with the help of a stick of *palāśa* (*Butea monosperma* Kuntze). This *nāga* (lead) should be added to the molten *bīja* for three times. Thus, the *bīja* becomes coloured and this should be used for the *rañjana saṃskāra* of mercury.

For *rañjana saṃskāra,* the *bīja* should be taken 1/64th in quantity of mercury in a *tapta khalva,* (heated mortar and pestle) and triturated for one day. Then it should be cooked in *Kacchapa yantra* (see App. II). According to the rules prescribed *in grāsa māna saṃskāra* the quantity of *bīja* should be increased gradually till it reaches six times of mercury.

SĀRAṆĀ SAṂSKĀRA (POTENTISATION)

Even after *jāraṇa* and *rañjana saṃskāras,* the potency of mercury is not adequate for *lauha siddhi* and *deha siddhi.* To make it adequately potent it is necessary that this mercury, after *rañjana saṃskāra* should undergo *sāraṇa saṃskāra.* For this purpose, a separate type of *bīja* called *vajra bīja* is needed. To make this *bīja* easily assimilable with mercury, a special type of medicated oil is necessary. This medicated oil is called *Sāraṇa taila.*

Preparation of Sāraṇa Taila

For the preparation of *Sāraṇa taila,* fat of either frog, fish, tortoise, sheep, leech, snake or pig should be collected. The oil of *jyotiṣmatī* (*Celastrus paniculatus* Willd.), *bibhītaka* (*Terminalia belerica* Roxb.), *karañja* (*Pongamia pinnata* Merr.) or *kaṭu tumbī* (*Lagenaria siceraria* Standl.) is used in this preparation. One part of the oil should be added with two parts of the decoction of drugs belonging to *rakta varga* (see description below) and four parts of milk. This should be cooked by adding 1/16th in quantity of the paste of *vidruma* (coral), *mañjiṣṭhā* (*Rubia cordifolia* Linn.), *lākṣā* (lac), *bhū nāga* (earth worm), stool of flies, crow or *śalabha* (grass hopper) and the ear-wax of buffalo. To this, one part of the above mentioned animal fat should be added while cooking. When properly cooked, it should be filtered and kept in a container. Some physicians prefer to add the paste of drugs belonging to *dvandva melāpana varga* (described below) to the above mentioned paste for quicker results.

Rakta Varga

Flowers of *dāḍima* (*Punica granatum* Linn.), *palāśa* (*Butea monosperma* Kuntze) and *bandhuka* (*Pentapetes phoenicea* Linn.), *rajanī* (*Curcuma longa* Linn.), *mañjiṣṭhā* (*Rubia cordifolia* Linn.), *lākṣā* (lac) and *rakta candana* (*Pterocarpus santalinus* Linn. f.)-- these drugs taken together are called *rakta varga.*

Dvandva Melāpana Varga

Ūrṇā (wool), *ṭaṅkaṇa* (borax), *śilā jatu* (mineral pitch), *indra gopa (Mutella occidentalis)* and *karkaṭaka* (crab)--all these taken together are called *dvandva melāpana varga.*

Preparation of Vajra Bīja

Twelve parts of gold, six parts of purified mercury, three parts of *nāga bhasma* (lead) and four parts of *pavi bhasma* (diamond)--all these four should be mixed together and triturated in a *tapta khalva* (hot mortar and pestle) by adding lemon juice. Trituration should be continued for twelve hours and then dried. It should then be kept inside a special type of crucible called *dvandva melāpana mūṣā* (see App. II). It should be sealed and kept over strong fire. This fire should be inflammed with the help of a blower for about six hours. All these four drugs then get mixed up and the compound is called *Vajra bīja.*

In a big size *gostanī mūṣā* (see App. II), *Sāraṇā oil* should be filled upto half of its capacity. The oil should be heated by placing the *mūṣā* over an oven. Inside the oil, mercury and *biḍa,* the latter 1/4th in quantity of the former, should be kept. The mouth of the *mūṣā* should be covered with a cloth. In a separate iron pan, *vajra bīja* which is taken in equal quantity (to that of mercury) is melted. This molten *bīja* is slowly poured over the cloth so that it goes inside *Sāraṇa taila* kept there. When the molten *vajra bīja* is poured over *Sāraṇa taila* it is likely to come out splashing when it comes into contact with the oil. The cloth covering the mouth of the *mūṣā* will prevent it. However, to prevent any accident, molten *bīja* should be poured very slowly and the physician should be at a comfortable distance. This would be possible if the iron pan used for melting the *bīja* has a long handle.

PRATI SĀRAṆA AND ANU SĀRAṆA

Sāraṇa is of three types. The first variety is called only *sāraṇa* without any epithet or prefix. The second variety is called *prati sāraṇa* and third variety is called *anu sāraṇa.* Even though similar processes are followed in these three types of *sāraṇa,* some physicians describe them as three different *saṃskāras.* Others, however, consider *prati sāraṇā* and *anu sāraṇā* as the two subsequent stages of *sāraṇā,* and include them under *sāraṇā saṃskāra.* In *sāraṇā,* equal quantity of *vajra bīja* was used, but in *prati sāraṇā, vajra bīja* should be used in double the quantity of mercury. In *anu sāraṇā,* the quantity of *vajra bīja* should be three times of mercury. This is the only difference. The procedure to be followed for both *prati sāraṇā* and *anu sāraṇā* is the same as the one prescribed for *sāraṇā.*

To prevent splashing during this *saṃskāra,* some physicians follow a slightly different method. Another funnel type *mūṣā* called *dhustūra puṣpa mūṣā* (see App. II) is prepared and kept over the *gostanī mūṣā.* The joint of both these *mūṣās* should be properly sealed. Through this funnel shaped *mūṣā* the molten metal should be poured. This ensures prevention of splashing.

In *sāraṇā, prati sāraṇā* and *anu sāraṇā,* small quantities of *nāga bhasma* (1/64th in quantity of mercury) should be added if *lauha siddhi* is to be achieved.

By *sāraṇā,* the mercury becomes enough potent to cause *vedha* (transmutation of mercury into gold) of one hundred times of mercury. By *prati sāraṇā,* it could cause *vedha* of one thousand times of mercury and by *anu sāraṇā* it becomes potent to cause *vedha* of ten thousand times of mercury. Exact implications of the term *vedha* will be explained later. This process of *anu sāraṇā* can be repeated, and every time the mercury becomes ten times more potent. Since this is an important *saṃskāra* for increasing the potency of mercury, and since it is difficult to be achieved, some physicians adopt a slightly different method for this purpose.

As before, a funnel shaped crucible *(dhustūra puṣpa mūṣā)* is prepared. Its tappering end should be eight *aṅgulas* (six inches) in length and its mouth should be four *aṅgulas* (three inches) in diameter. The mouth of this *mūṣā* should be closed. Over this, another crucible (same type) is kept with its mouth upwards. There should be a hole at the bottom of the upper crucible. The joints between these two *mūṣās* should be properly sealed. Through the upper crucible mercury should be poured which will come down to the lower crucible through the hole made at the bottom of the upper one. Through the upper crucible, again *Sāraṇā taila* mixed with the paste of the stool of *bhū nāga* (earthworm), *kāka* (crow) or *pataṅga* (grass hopper), honey and ear-wax of baffalo (each 1/16th in quantity of mercury) should be added. *Sāraṇā taila* should be filled half of the capacity of the upper crucible in addition to the lower one. In the upper *mūṣā,* the *bīja* mixed with the above paste should be kept. The mouth of the upper crucible should be covered with a lid and the joint should be sealed with seven layers of mud smeared cloth (the mud should be mixed with 1/4th in quantity of rock-salt).

After the seal is dried up, both these crucibles should be placed in a pit dug into the earth so that 3/4th of the upper crucible remains inside it and only 1/4th remains projecting outside. Over this, strong heat should be employed by charcoal or cow-dung cake fuel. The fire should be inflammed with the help of a blower. This will help in melting the *bīja* and through *Sāraṇā taila* it will go to the lower crucible. There, it will get mixed up with mercury. The proces is facilitated and expedited if *biḍa* or catalytic agent (see App. I) 1/64th in quantity of mercury is added to it.

KRĀMAṆA SAṂSKĀRA (PENETRATION)

The term *krāmaṇa* literally means 'penetration'. By this *saṃskāra* mercury becomes capable of entering into each and every tissue element in the body (in respect of *deha siddhi*) and each and every atom of the metal (in respect of *lauha siddhi*). Without *krāmaṇa saṃskāra,* mercury becomes incapable of converting the base metals into noble metals like gold and silver; it only imparts colour to the exterior of the metal which is practically of no significance. As the food and drinks after digestion and metabolism pervade all the tissues of the body, similarly by *krāmaṇa saṃskāra* mercury becomes capable of entering into each and every tissue cells of the body and each and every atom of the metal.

Several recipes have been described for *krāmaṇa saṃskāra.* Some of them are common to both *deha siddhi* and *lauha siddhi.* But some others are specific either for *deha siddhi* or for *lauha siddhi. Kānta* (magnetic iron) *bhasma, viṣa* (aconite), *rasaka* (calamine), *hiṅgula* (cinnabar) and *indra gopa* (*Mutella occidentalis*) should be mixed with *Rañjana taila* (described before) and made to a paste. This paste should be applied over mercury and cooked by *gaja puṭa* (see App. II). If the intention is to prepare gold out of base metals then the *bhasma* of *nāga* (lead) prepared by adding *manaḥ śīlā* (realgar) should be added to the paste. *Nāga bhasma* should be 1/64th in quantity of mercury.

If the intention is to prepare silver out of base metals, then *bhasma* of *vaṅga* (tin) prepared by adding *tālaka* (orpiment) should be mixed with the paste. The *bhasma* of *nāga* or *vaṅga* should be added to the paste and triturated by adding lemon juice. These two recipes are for *lauha siddhi.* For *deha siddhi* some more *bhasma* of *kānta lauha* (1/64th in quantity of mercury) should be added to the paste and further triturated by adding lemon juice. In all these recipes, addition of the *sattva* of *mākṣika* or copper pyrite (1/64th in quantity of mercury) will be advantageous.

Krāmaṇa saṃskāra is actually performed along with *vedha saṃskāra* which is being described below.

VEDHA SAMSKĀRA (TARNSMUTATION)

Vedha saṃskāra is of four types, viz. (1) *lepa vedha,* (2) *kṣepa vedha,* (3) *kunta vedha,* and (4) *dhūma vedha.* The paste of drugs described for *krāmaṇa saṃskāra* should be applied over the base metal and further processed. This is called *lepa vedha.* The base metal is reduced to its liquid state by heating *(biḍa* has to be added during this process). To this molten metal, processed mercury along with the paste described in *krāmaṇa saṃskāra* should be added. This is called *kṣepa vedha.* If the processed mercury along with the paste of drugs is taken in a spoon and immersed suddenly into the molten metal, then it is called *kunta vedha.* If over the burnt charcoal having smoke, mercury and the prescribed paste are kept, and to this smoke, the base metal is exposed for its transmutation to noble metal, then this is called *dhūma vedha.* In this process, mercury and paste are kept inside the mouth of a person who blows over the base metal for its transmutation.

Hemākṛṣṭi

Mercury (one part), *hiṅgula* or cinnabar (two parts), *sattva* of *svarṇa mākṣika* or chalco pyrite (three parts), *gandhaka* or sulphur (four parts) and *manaḥ śilā* or realgar (five parts) should be made to a paste and applied over thin plates of copper. Then with the help of the juice of *cāṅgerī* (*Oxalis corniculata* Linn.), it should be impregnated and triturated. After drying, it should be cooked in *gaja puṭa.* This should be repeated for five times. The *bhasma,* thus prepared, should be immersed in molten lead. This is called *hemākṛṣṭi.* This powder is used for transmutation of base metals into gold.

Several other methods have been described for transmutation of base metals into gold. For example, ninety eight parts of silver, one part of mercury (collected from previous *saṃskāra*) and one part of gold should be mixed with the paste of drugs described in *krāmaṇa saṃskāra.* This should be cooked in *kapota puṭa* (see App. II). This converts the whole compound into gold.

Forty-nine parts of silver, forty-nine parts of copper, one part of gold and one part of mercury (collected after *krāmaṇa saṃskāra*) should be added with the paste of drugs described *in krāmaṇa saṃskāra* and cooked in *kapota puṭa.* This converts the whole compound into gold.

In the above mentioned examples, only *śata vedhī* (transmutation of hundred times) method has been described in which one part of processed mercury can cause transmutation of ninety-nine parts of other metals into gold. After *prati sāraṇa* and *anu sāraṇa*, described before, processed mercury becomes more potent and it can cause transmutation of one thousand, ten thousand and even ten million times of base metals into gold.

Tārākṛṣṭi

Bhasma of *vaṅga* (tin) should be added with equal quantity of *tāmra* (copper) and melted over fire. To this, one hundredth part of processed mercury and equal quantity of *tālaka* (orpiment) should be added. The latter should be added in small instalments and triturated by keeping the compound in a *tapta khalva*. This compound should be kept in a *mūṣā* (crucible) and made to melt. Thereafter, the *bhasma* of *nāga* (lead) should be added to it. To this, *tāla* (orpiment), *śilā* (realgar), *svarji kṣāra* (Sodium bicarbonate), *saindhava lavaṇa* (rock-salt) and the *bhasma* of *kharpara* (calamine)-- all taken in quantity equal to that of the molten compound -- should be added.

The crucible should be strongly heated till the whole compound melts. This molten compound should be immersed in the solution of cow-dung. This process should be repeated and the molten metal should be immersed in butter-milk, latex of *snuhī* (*Euphorbia neriifolia* Linn.), ghee, solution of jaggery, milk and honey--once in each. To this, *sattva* of *raupya mākṣika* (iron pyrite), *pittala* (brass), *vaṅga* (tin) and *sattva* of *tāla* (orpiment) -- all taken in equal quantity should be added and cooked in a crucible over strong fire till it melts. If this compound is added to one hundred times of the base metal, then the latter gets transmutated into pure silver. This process is called *tārākṛṣṭi*.

KṢETRĪ KARAṆA (PROCESSING THE BODY)

In some ayurvedic texts, this is treated as one of the *saṃskāras*. It is the process of making the body of the individual suitable for the administration of processed mercury for the purpose of rejuvenation and for *sadeha mukti* (attaining salvation while alive).

Before administering the processed mercury to a person, it is necessary that his body should be made suitable for this purpose. As it is not possible to properly paint a picture over a dirty canvas, similarly, a dirty body containing a lot of metabolic waste products will not be suitable to accept and utilize the processed mercury for the purpose of rejuvenation and for curing obstinate diseases. Several methods have been described in ayurvedic texts for cleansing the body. Several recipes are also prescribed in ayurvedic texts to be used for a limited period.

There are five special therapies which are administered according to a prescribed method for cleansing the body. These therapies, taken together, are called *pañca karma* (five therapies).

Generally, *pañca karma* includes *vamana* (emetic therapy), *virecana* (purgation therapy), *nirūha basti* (medicated enema prepared of decoctions, etc.), *anuvāsana basti* (medicated enema prepared of oil, etc.) and *nasya* (inhalation therapy). Prior to this *pañca karma* therapy, *snehana* (oleation therapy) and *svedana* (fomentation therapy) are administered. These are only preparatory measures (*pūrva karma*).

In the present context, however, *pañca karma* includes *pācana* therapy (drugs to stimulate the power of digestion and metabolism), *snehana* (oleation therapy), *svedana* (fomentation therapy), *vamana* (emetic therapy) and *virecana* (purgation therapy). Several recipes have been described for these purposes.

Pācana Therapy

Before the administration of this therapy, the patient should use light diet during the day time. One *pala* (48 gm.) of each of *kṣudrā* (*Solanum xanthocarpum* Schrad & Wendl), *dhānyaka* (*Coriandrum sativum* Linn.) and *nāgara* (*Zingiber officinale* Rosc.) should be boiled by adding eight times of water and reduced to 1/8th. This should be filtered and the decoction should be taken at night for three consecutive days. Thereafter, the decoction of *triphalā* (a collective name for *harītakī* or *Terminalia chebula* Retz., *bibhītakī* or *Terminalia belerica* Roxb., and *āmalakī* or *Emblica officinalis* Gaertn.) taken in the same quantity and processed according to the same method should be taken at night for three consecutive nights.

Snehana (Oleation) Therapy

During day time the individual should take rice and ghee mixed with the soup of goat meat (for non-vegetarians) or the soup of *mudga* or *Phaseolus mungo* Linn. (for vegetarians). The quantity of rice should be such as will be easily digestible during the day time. At night the patient should be given cow's ghee (4 *niṣkas* or 12 gm.) mixed with rock-salt (one *niṣka* or 3 gm.). This should be given consecutively for seven days. During day time, massage should be done with the help of *Bhṛṅgāmalaka taila*.

Svedana (Fomentation) Therapy

In an earthen pot, *māṣa* (*Phaseolus radiatus* Linn.), *tila* (*Sesamum indicum* Linn.), *yava* (*Hordeum vulgare* Linn.), *āmalaka* (*Emblica officinalis* Gaertn.) and *saktu* (roasted corn flour) (all one *prastha* or seven hundred seventy gms. in quantity), *agaru* (*Aquilaria agallocha* Roxb.), *balā* (*Sida cordifolia* Linn.), *rāsnā* (*Pluchea lanceolata* Oliver & Hiern.), *vyāghrī* (*Solanum xanthocarpum* Schrad and Wendle.), *dhānā* (fried paddy), *patra* (*Cinnamomum tamala* Nees. and Eberm.), *kauśika* (*Commiphora mukul* Engl.), *ativiṣā* (*Aconitum heterophyllum* Wall.) and *niśā* (*Curcuma longa* Linn.) -- all two *palas* or 96 gms. in quantity-should be taken. To this, two *āḍhakas* (6 Ltrs.) of butter-milk, milk, water and *kāñjī* (vinegar) should be added and boiled. With the steam of these drugs, fomentation therapy should be administered. For this purpose, a special type of equipment has to be used.

The patient should sleep over a bed. The lower portion of the bed should be closed. A heater or stove should be kept in this lower chamber and the mud pot containing the above mentioned drugs should be boiled over this heater. The plank of the bed should have holes for the steam to come from the lower chamber to the upper chamber. The bed should be covered with a blanket and the patient should sleep over it. The patient should be covered with another blanket. The steam will thus circulate between these two blankets and the patient will get fomented. Fomentation should not be applied to the head of the patient. Throughout the fomentation therapy, the head of the patient should rest over a pillow and it should not be covered. The fomentation therapy should be applied for two hours every day in the early morning. The patient should be in empty stomach during this therapy. This should be done consecutively for seven days.

Vamana (Emetic) Therapy

One *tolā* (12 gm.) of *madana* (*Randia dumetorum* Lam.) should be added with equal quantity of the root of *pāṭhā* (*Cissampelos pareira* Linn.). To this, thirty two *tolās* of water should be added and boiled till 1/4th remains. This should be strained through a cloth. To this decoction, the powder of *pippalī* (*Piper longum* Linn.), *indra yava* (*Holarrhena antidysenterica* Wall.), *yaṣṭī* (*Glycyrrhiza glabra* Linn.) and *saindhava* (rock-salt)-- one gm. of each--should be added. This should be given to the patient by which there will be vomiting. If properly conducted, one day therapy will be enough. At the end of the vomiting, bile should come out. If this does not happen then the emetic therapy should be repeated for the second or third day also.

Virecana (Purgation) Therapy

Purified mercury, *bhasma* of *ṭaṅkaṇa* (borax), purified sulphur, *trikaṭu* (collective name for *pippalī* or *Piper longum* Linn., *marica* or *Piper nigrum* Linn. and *śuṇṭhī* or *Zingiber officinalis* Rosc.) and *triphalā* (collective name for *harītakī* or *Terminalia chebula* Retz., *bibhītakī* or *Terminalia belerica* Roxb. and *āmalakī* or *Emblica officinalis* Gaertn.)—one part of each—and nine parts of *jaya pāla* (*Croton tinglium* Linn.) should be triturated till a thin paste is made out. Pills of 250 mg. each should be prepared out of this paste. One of these pills should be given to the patient along with one *tolā* (12 gm.) of jaggery early in the morning in empty stomach with a cup of warm water. Before adding to the recipe, *jaya pāla* should be purified according to the prescribed procedure. The patient, thereafter, will start purging and at the end of it, *kapha* or phlegm will come out. The therapy for one day will be enough for the purpose. But if *kapha* or phlegm does not come out then the therapy should be repeated for the second or third day also.

Correction of the Residual Doṣas

After *pañca karma* therapy, it is necessary to correct some of the residual *doṣas* which are the metabolic by-products in the form of excess salts, alkalies and acids or infective organisms (*kṛmis*). To correct these defects, following remedies should be employed:

Correction of Excessive Salts

The individual should be given one *kuḍava* (192 ml.) of the juice of the stilt-root of *ketakī* (*Pandanus tectorius* Soland. ex Parkinson) and *jambīra* (*Citrus limon* Burm. f.) for seven days. This potion should be administered every day early in the morning. This corrects excessive salts in the body.

Correction of Excessive Alkalies

One *pala* (48 gms.) of *triphalā* (collective name for *harītakī* or *Terminalia chebula* Retz., *bibhītakī* or *Terminalia belerica* Roxb., and *āmalakī* or *Emblica officinalis* Gaertn.) should be boiled in sixteen *palas* of water and reduced to 1/4th. After filtering, this decoction should be mixed with one *pala* of honey and given to the patient early in the morning for consecutively three days. This corrects excessive alkalies in the body.

Correction of Excessive Acids

The decoction of *viḍaṅga* (*Embelia ribes* Burm. f.), *vāsā* (*Adhatoda vasica* Nees.), *kuṣṭha* (*Saussurea lappa* C.B. Clarke) and *ketakī* (*Pandanus tectorius* Soland. ex Parkinson) should be given to the patient consecutively for three days. This corrects excessive *amla* (acids) in the body. For the preparation of this decoction, one *pala* (48 gms.) of drugs should be boiled in sixteen *palas* of water and reduced to 1/4th.

Removal of Parasites

One *karṣa* (12 gms.) of each of *vāsā* (*Adhatoda vasica* Nees.), *viḍaṅga* (*Embelia ribes* Burm. f.) and seed of *palāśa* (*Butea monosperma* Kuntze) should be added with one *karṣa* of jaggery and administered to the individual with hot water. It should be given in powder form in the morning for consecutively three days. This helps in the removal of infective organisms from the body.

Correction of Residual Doṣas

In spite of the above mentioned regimens and remedies, some *doṣas* may still remain inside the body. To remove these *doṣas,* one *karṣa* (12 gms.) of the powder of *śyāmā (Operculina turpethum* Silva Manso), *vahni* (*Plumbago zeylanica* Linn.), *viḍaṅga* (*Embelia ribes* Burm. f.), *vāsā* (*Adhatoda vasica* Nees), *trikaṭu* (collective name of *śuṇṭhī* or *Zingiber officinalis* Rosc., *pippalī* or *Piper longum* Linn. and *marica* or *Piper nigrum* Linn.), *triphalā* (collective name for *harītakī* or *Terminalia chebula* Retz., *bibhītakī* or *Teriminalia belerica* Roxb. and *āmalakī* or *Emblica officinalis* Gaertn.), *saindhava* (rock-salt), *devadāru* (*Cedrus deodara* Loud.) and *mustā* (*Cyperus rotundus* Linn.)-- all taken in equal quantities, should be mixed with ghee and made to a linctus. This should be given to the person consecutively for seven days.

Revival of Strength

Because of the above mentioned therapies, the person will become physically weak. Therefore, after the purification of the body he should be made to eat *śālī* (a variety of *Oryza sativa* Linn.) types of rice along with milk till he regains his full strength. Thereafter, processed mercury should be administered for the purpose of rejuvenation.

ADMINISTRATION OF MERCURY

Mercury, which has been processed according to the method described above, should now be administered to the person for the purpose of rejuvenation. The previous *saṃskāra* i.e. *lauha siddhi* is done simply to test the potency of mercury. In fact for the purpose of rejuvenation, *āroṭa* type of mercury can be administered to the person. Mercury, after *rañjana saṃskāra* is called *āroṭa*. This can be used alone or in combination with some other drugs. Generally, *kānta loha* (magnetic iron) *bhasma* and *bhasma* of *abhraka* (mica) *sattva* are added to the *āroṭa* type of mercury and administered. All these three should be taken in equal quantities and administered in the dose of two *guñjās* (one *guñjā*=125 mg.). This should be mixed with honey and ghee (in unequal quantity, approximately two tea spoons) and given to the person early in the morning for continuously two months. Thereafter, the dose should be increased by one *guñjā* (125 mg.) and given to the patient for one month. Subsequently, every month, the dose should be increased by one *guñjā* (125 mg.) and given to the patient in total for sixteen months. The person who has taken processed mercury for sixteen months in the above mentioned manner will live for full span of life without wrinkles in his face and without greying of hair in his head.

Several other recipes are described in ayurvedic texts for the purpose of rejuvenation. Scholars interested in these details may refer to any standard ayurvedic text specially on *rasa śāstra*. Some of them are meant for promoting excessive virility (aphrodisiac therapy) and some others are for attaining super-natural powers like flying in the sky, etc. The ultimate aim of using processed mercury is to make the body and the mind of the individual absolutely clean by which he leads an unblemished life of *jīvan mukta* (salvation while living in the physical body). Several recipes and methods have been described to attain this state of *jīvan mukti*, and to make the body as well as the mind pure. These are not being described here.

For attaining the state of *jīvan mukti*, mercury therapy may, if necessary, be supplemented with yogic practices. The person who has used processed mercury can practice several yogic methods and acquire super-natural powers which taken together are called *aṣṭa siddhi*, viz. *aṇimā* (subtlety), *mahimā* (unlimited expansion), *laghimā* (excessive lightness), *garimā* (excessive heaviness), *prāptī* (ability to acquire anything he desires), *prākāmya* (unlimited strength), *īśitva* (omnipotence) and *vaśitva* (acquiring the power to control all physical and natural phenomena).

While using processed mercury, the person has to observe several dos and don'ts and he has to lead a disciplined life. His food and drinks are to be regulated and he has to adopt certain regimens. Details of all these can be found in standard texts on *Rasa śāstra* (Iatro-chemistry). If these regimens are not followed strictly then the person will not only lose all good effects of the therapy but the therapy may give rise to several complications. The method of the management of these complications and correction of the resultant morbidities are described in detail in ayurvedic texts.

CHAPTER-V

POPULARLY USED MERCURIAL PREPARATIONS

PREPARATIONS OF MERCURY

Several thousands of mercurial preparations are used in ayurvedic practice. By way of illustrations, a few of these commonly used compounds are being discussed here. For these preparations the most effective would be mercury processed according to the eighteen *saṃskāras* described before. Since this involves difficult process, since the description in respect of these processes is cryptic, since there are very few adepts in these methods and since these saints often do not want to impart this knowledge for fear of its misuse by unscrupulous persons, generally mercury of the following types are used in most of these preparations, and obviously, these are not as effective as the textual claims in respect of these preparations are made.

1. Mercury processed according to the first eight *saṃskāras;*
2. Mercury collected from *hiṅgula* by distillation; and
3. Mercury processed according to simpler methods.

Of course, textual quotations are cited to justify the use of such easy methods. But such quotations, particularly in respect of the last two methods described above, according to some scholars, are spurious and subsequent interpolations. By these methods, no doubt, mercury is made non-toxic. Therapeutically, the first variety is more effective than the subsequent two varieties. Aṣṭa *saṃskāras* (first eight *saṃskāras*) of mercury are already described. The remaining two methods are described below in brief.

Collection of Mercury from Cinnabar

Hiṅgula (cinnabar) should be impregnated by adding lemon juice and triturated for three hours in a mortar and pestle. From out of this paste, circular and flat lumps (of about one inch diameter) should be prepared and dried in the sun. These lumps should be kept in a *tiryak pātana yantra* (see App. II) and by the method of distillation, mercury should be collected. This mercury should be cooked in *dolā yantra* (see App. II) by adding *kāñjī* (a type of vinegar) for six hours. Then it should be washed with hot water. The mercury, thus collected, is used in medicine.

Simpler Methods for Processing Mercury

Mercury should be mixed with equal quantity of lime powder and triturated for three days. Then, through a cloth mercury should be strained out. To this mercury, equal quantity of garlic paste with half the quantity of rock-salt should be added and triturated till the garlic paste becomes black in colour. It needs about six hours of trituration. Thereafter, mercury should be collected by washing with *kāñjī* (a type of vinegar). The mercury, thus collected, is used in medicinal preparations.

Mūrchana

To make mercury processed according to the above mentioned three methods, effective in the treatment of diseases, it is further processed which is called *mūrcchana*. It is necessary to clarify here that this *mūrchana* is different from the *mūrchana saṃskāra* (the third process) described before. *Mūrchana* is of two types, viz., (1) *sagandha mūrchana* and (2) *nirgandha mūrchana*. In the former, sulphur is added to mercury and the latter is performed by adding different drugs (other than sulphur). Preparations of the former category are harmless. These are populary used for curing various types of diseases and for the purpose of rejuvenation as well as promotion of virility. These preparations can be used for a long period.

On the other hand, preparations of the latter category (which are prepared without adding sulphur) are toxic. These are generally used for curing some obstinate diseases and discontinued after the prescribed course or when the disease is cured, whichever is earlier. Rarely, these drugs are used for rejuvenation purposes. Important preparations of the former category are *Kajjalī*, *Rasa parpaṭī*, *Rasa sindūra* and *Makara dhvaja*. Preparations of the latter category are *Rasa puṣpa*, *Rasa karpūra* and *Mugdha rasa*.

Bahirdhūma and Antardhūma Methods

Sagandha mūrcchana is of two types, viz., (1) *bahirdhūma mūrchana* and (2) *antardhūma mūrchana*. In the former, cooking is done while exposing the ingredients to external air, and in the latter, cooking is done without exposure to air. *Bahirdhūma* method is followed for the preparation of several commonly used ayurvedic medicines. *Antardhūma* method is followed only for some special preparations like special varieties of *Rasa sindūra* and *Makara dhvaja*.

KAJJALĪ

In a *khalva* (mortar and pestle) made of iron or stone, purified mercury and sulphur should be taken in equal quantities and triturated. Gradually the white colour of mercury and the yellow colour of sulphur will disappear and a black powder will be formed. This should be further triturated till the powder becomes very fine like collyrium *(kajjalī)* and the dazzling particles of mercury completely disappear. At this stage of trituration, it will be better to sprinkle a few drops of water over the powder to prevent spilling. This is the general method. In different medicines, purified mercury and purified sulphur are mixed in different proportions.

Testing

After completion of the process, *kajjalī* should be tested to ascertain its suitability for therapeutic purposes. Some particles of *kajjalī* should be placed over gold and rubbed by adding a drop of lemon juice. If mercury particles remain separate from sulphur particles (which may not be ordinarily visible to the naked eye), then there will be a white line like silver over the gold. If it so happens then the process of trituration should be continued further.

Kajjalī as such is at times used externally. Internally, it is seldom used alone in ayurvedic practice. Generally for internal purpose, it is used in combination with other drugs in a recipe. If in the recipe, the ratio of mercury and sulphur is not indicated, then both these ingredients are to be taken in equal quantities. In some recipes these two ingredients are specified to be used in a different proportion. In such cases, *kajjalī* should be prepared by taking these two ingredients in the specified quantities.

RASA PARPAṬĪ (SCALE PREPARATION)

The method of purification of mercury is already described. The method of purification of sulphur will be described later. But for the preparation of *parpaṭī,* mercury and sulphur are to be processed in a specific manner. Mercury (already processed according to eight *saṃskāras)* should be impregnated and triturated by adding the juice of *bhṛṅga rāja (Eclipta alba* Hassk.), *jayā* (*Sesbania bispinosa* Fawcett & Rendle), *eraṇḍa* (*Ricinus communis* Linn.) and *kāka mācī (Solanum nigrum* Linn.), for one day in each. Sulphur should be made to a coarse powder and triturated by adding the juice of *bhṛṅga rāja* (*Eclipta alba* Hassk.) for three days. In an iron pan smeared with ghee, this sulphur should be kept and the iron pan should be placed over an oven with mild fire. It will melt gradually. In another pot, juice of *bhṛṅga rāja* (*Eclipta alba* Hassk.) should be kept upto half of its capacity and its mouth should be covered with a piece of cloth which should be tied properly. Over this cloth, the melted sulphur should be slowly poured. When this liquid sulphur will come in contact with the juice of *bhṛṅga rāja,* sulphur will solidify again. This should then be removed from the pot, washed with hot water and dried. Mercury and sulphur, thus processed, should be made to a *kajjalī* by triturating in a mortar and pestle. To prevent its spilling, at the last stage, drops of water should be sprinkled over the powder while triturating.

When the *kajjalī* is prepared, it should be kept in an iron spoon smeared with ghee. Over the oven, iron pan should be kept. It should be covered with a layer of sand of about 3/4th" in thickness. Over this sand, the iron spoon containing *kajjalī* (powder of mercury and sulphur) should be kept. The purpose of keeping sand over the iron pan is to provide slow but continuous heat to *kajjalī*. Because of the heat, *kajjalī* will gradually melt. To bring uniformity in melting, it is necessary to stir the compound periodically with the help of a spatula.

In the meantime, over a smooth and even surface, cow-dung should be spread, about one inch in thickness and six inches in diameter. Over it, an intact banana-leaf should be kept. The melted *kajjalī* should be poured over the smooth surface of the banana-leaf. Over this, another banana-leaf should be placed covered with a layer of cow-dung. From the above, gentle pressure should be applied. Because of the cold touch of the banana-leaf and cow-dung, the melted *kajjalī* will solidify and because of pressure, it will take flat shape like a thin scale. This is called *Rasa parpaṭī*.

Cooking of *parpaṭī* is of three types, viz., (1) *mṛdu pāka* (mild cooking), (2) *madhya pāka* (moderate cooking) and (3) *khara pāka* (over-cooking). These modes of cooking are tested by breaking the scale preparation. If while breaking, it bends, then it is mild cooking. If it breaks into small pieces without bending, then it is moderate cooking. If it is reduced to powder by applying pressure, then it is over-cooking. The second type is the best for therapeutic purposes. The first variety will be therapeutically less effective. But the over-cooked (*khara pāka*) *parpaṭī* is harmful and it should never be used in medicine.

Dosage

Rasa parpaṭī is administered to a patient in a gradually increased dose. On the first day, it is administered in the dose of 125 mg. (one *rattī*). It should be increased on subsequent days by 125 mg. per day for nine days more. This dose of 125 mg. per day should be continued till the patient is relieved of his ailments. This total amount of 1250 mg. can be given in a single dose or two or three divided doses. Generally, this optimum dose is continued for twenty days and then it is reduced by 125 mg. each subsequent days. Thus, the complete course is for forty days. This course can be altered depending upon the response of the patient. If the disease is cured earlier or if the patient shows any toxic manifestation, it should be terminated earlier and discontinued by tappering off. If, however, the patient is not cured of his ailment, the course can be repeated by a gap of about seven days. This type of giving medicine in a gradually increased and decreased dose is called *kalpa*. In respect of *parpaṭī* it is called *parpaṭī kalpa*.

Apart from this *kalpa* therapy, *parpaṭī* can also be given routinely in a dose of 125 mg. twice daily in empty stomach.

Other Forms of Parpaṭī

To make it therapeutically more potent and more specific in curing an ailment, it is added with different other ingredients like the *bhasma* of gold, copper, iron, etc., and accordingly these *parpaṭīs* are called *svarṇa parpaṭī, tāmra parpaṭī, lauha parpaṭī, pañcāmṛta parpaṭī*, etc. For their administration, the same method as described for *Rasa parpaṭī* is followed.

Anupāna or Vehicle

Parpaṭī should be administered with three gm. of the powder of cumin seeds and fifty mg. of the powder of asafoetida (which is processed by frying with ghee). *Parpaṭī* can also be administered with milk or cream.

Diet

The patient using *parpaṭī kalpa* should be kept only on milk, butter-milk or fruit juice. If found necessary, some rice can be given to the patient. But other cereals, pulses, salt and water are to be strictly prohibited. In view of the prohibition of water, *parpaṭī kalpa* is generally avoided in summer. In case of emergency, however, it can be given in summer with ample quantity of milk. By this drug, the patient becomes capable of digesting enormous quantity of milk. For better effect, he should be given cow's milk in preference to other types of milk. He can digest even twenty litres of milk per day even though, before treatment, he might have been very allergic to even a spoon of milk.

Other Regimens

The patient during the administration of *parpaṭī kalpa* should take rest and should not exert too much. Even after the course of *parpaṭī kalpa* is over, the patient should not resort to any strenuous work and should take only light diet for about three months.

Indications

Parpaṭī kalpa is useful in all the diseases of the gastro-intestinal tract. It is specially useful in the treatment of sprue syndrome, chronic colitis, chronic diarrhoea, *agni māndya* (suppression of the power of digestion) and serious types of *pāṇḍu* (anemia).

RASA SINDŪRA

Purified mercury (32 *tolās*), purified sulphur (16 *tolās*), *nava sādara* or Ammonium chloride (one *tolā* or 12 gm.) and *sphaṭika* or alulo (one *tolā*) should be triturated in a *khalva* (mortar and pestle) till *kajjalī* is formed. A strong glass bottle (generally used for packing alcoholic drinks) should be wrapped with seven layers of mud smeared cloth and dried. *Kajjalī* should be kept in this bottle. Care should be taken to see that the quantity of *kajjalī* should not exceed one third of the capacity of the glass bottle. This bottle should then be kept in a *Vālukā yantra* (see App. II). There should be a round hole, about one inch in diameter, at the bottom of the pot of this *yantra*. Over this hole, a copper coin should be kept and upon it the glass bottle containing *kajjalī* of the above-mentioned drugs should be placed erect. The remaining space in the pot should be filled with sand. The pot of *Vālukā yantra* should be placed over the oven and gradually mild, moderate and strong heat should be applied.

Mild heat should be employed for the first six hours. Because of heat, the fume of sulphur will come out from the mouth of the bottle. An iron rod with wooden handle should be heated by keeping inside the oven and this red hot iron should be periodically inserted into the mouth of the bottle to keep it clean of sulphur deposits. Thereafter, moderate heat should be employed and the heat should be gradually increased. In the beginning, sulphur particles will stick to the hot iron rod when it is inserted into the glass bottle. But when all the sulphur is consumed, then there will be no sulphur fume and no sulphur will stick to the inserted iron rod.

At this stage, if carefully peeped through the mouth of the bottle, its bottom will appear red. This is the time when the mouth of the bottle should be closed with a cork made out of a piece of brick and it should be properly sealed with the help of a mud-smeared cloth. The mud for this purpose should be mixed with a small quantity of lime and jaggery. Then for the next six hours strong heat should be employed. Thereafter, the *Vālukā yantra* including the glass bottle should be allowed to cool down of its own.

The bottle should then be removed from the sand and the mud smeared cloth should be scrapped out through a knife. A thread or a cotton tape smeared in kerosene should be tied around the bottle and ignited. When the bottle is still hot, cold water should be poured over it. This will result in the cracking of the bottle. Then carefully crystallized *Rasa sindūra* deposited at the neck of the bottle should be removed with the help of a knife. The bottle should not be broken by pressure because in that case the broken pieces of glass might get mixed up with *Rasa sindūra*. It will be difficult to separate these glass pieces from crystals of *Rasa sindūra* at a later stage. These crystals should then be triturated in a *khalva* (mortar and pestle) for three days and made to a fine powder. This is used in the treatment of diseases and for rejuvenation purposes either alone or in combination with other drugs.

Dosage

125 to 250 mg. per day in a single or in two divided doses.

Anupāna or Vehicle

Generally honey is used as *anupāna* for *Rasa sindūra.* But for the treatment of various diseases different types of *anupāna* are prescribed in ayurvedic texts. Milk or cream should be used as *anupāna* if it is summer season or if the drug produces heating effect in the body.

Indications

Rasa sindūra is promoter of strength. It is aphrodisiac and *yoga-vāhin* (which potentiates and enhances the therapeutic efficacy of other drugs when added). It is extensively used for the purpose of *rasāyana* (rejuvenation). With different types of *anupānas,* it is useful in the treatment of several obstinate and otherwise incurable diseases.

TALASTHA RASA SINDŪRA

It has been described before that *sagandha mūrcchana* is of two types, viz., *bahirdhūma pāka* and *antardhūma pāka. Rasa sindūra* prepared according to *bahirdhūma pāka* method is already described. This recipe can also be prepared according to *antardhūma pāka* method which is called *Talastha rasa sindūra.*

For *Talastha rasa sindūra,* purified mercury and purified sulphur are mixed together and made to a *kajjalī* by triturating in a *khalva* (mortar and pestle). This *kajjalī* is kept in a bottle wrapped with seven layers of mud-smeared cloth. Its mouth (unlike the previous method of preparing *Rasa sindūra*) is sealed in the beginning itself. A pit (two feet in length, breadth and depth) should be dug in the earth. The sealed bottle should be kept at the centre of the pit and covered with about three inches of sand all around it. The remaining space in the pit should then be covered with cow-dung cakes and ignited. When it cools down, *Rasa sindūra* formed at the bottom of the bottle should be taken out by scrapping. This is called *Talastha rasa sindūra* and the method is called *antardhūma pāka.*

Ṣaḍguṇa Bali Jāraṇa

Even though *Rasa sindūra*, in general, is prepared by mixing equal quantities of mercury and sulphur, its more potent forms can be prepared by mixing two, three or even six times of sulphur. If while cooking, two parts of sulphur is added to mercury, then it is called *Dvi guṇa bali jārita rasa sindūra*. If three parts of sulphur is added to one part of mercury while cooking, then the *Rasa sindūra*, thus prepared, is called *Tri guṇa bali jārita*. Similarly, if six times of sulphur is added to mercury (one part) then it is called *Ṣaḍ guṇa bali jārita rasa sindūra*.

The term *jāraṇa*, used in the present context, has a different connotation from *jāraṇa* which is one of the eighteen *saṃskāras* of mercury. *Rasa sindūra* and *Makara dhvaja* (to be discussed latter) can be prepared according to this *Ṣaḍ guṇa bali jāraṇa* process. Other ingredients and method remaining the same, only sulphur is used six times in quantity of mercury during the process of preparing *kajjalī*. Some physicians follow a different method for this *Ṣaḍ guṇa bali jāraṇa*. They prepare *kajjalī* by mixing equal quantities of mercury and sulphur and *Rasa sindūra* is prepared. To this *Rasa sindūra*, another part of sulphur is added and triturated. From this powder, again *Rasa sindūra* is prepared. This process is repeated for four times more. Thus, final product is the outcome of six parts of sulphur.

MAKARA DHVAJA

In ayurvedic texts, several recipes have been described for the preparation of *Makara dhvaja*. The one commonly used in ayurvedic practice is being described here. Thirty-two *tolās* (one *tolā* = 12 gm.) of purified mercury should be kept in a mortar. To this, four *tolās* of leaves of purified gold should be added. Purification method of gold will be described later. These gold leaves are to be added to mercury one by one and triturated till it is properly amalgamated with the latter. To this, sixty four *tolās* of purified sulphur should be added and triturated. Thereafter, the juice of tender leaves and buds of banyan tree and the juice of *kumārī* (*Aloe barbadensis* Mill) should be added one after the other and triturated till a fine paste is formed.

The term *Makara dhvaja* is a synonym of Kāma deva, the god of sex. If *Makara dhvaja* is to be used for aphrodisiac purposes, then it is necessary that the *kajjalī* should be further impregnated by adding the juice of the red flower of cotton and triturated. After the *kajjalī* is dried, it should be kept in a glass bottle and cooked in *Vālukā yantra*. The preparation of the bottle and the method of cooking as described for *Rasa sindūra* adhering to the neck of the bottle should be collected by scrapping with the help of a knife. The powder of gold will remain at the bottom of the bottle.

This gold powder and the sublimed *Makara dhvaja* should be mixed and well triturated for three days. To this, the powder of *lavaṅga* (clove), *jātīphala* (nutmeg) and saffron, each half in quantity of *Makara dhvaja*, should be added and triturated by adding the juice of betel-leaf. This trituration should continue for at least three days. Thereafter, camphor and musk, each 1/8th in quantity of *Makara dhvaja* should be added and again triturated with the juice of the betel-leaf. From the paste, thus formed, pills should be made out, 250 mg. each. These pills should be dried in shade and kept in a glass bottle.

Doses

Two of the above mentioned pills should be given in the morning and two pills in the afternoon in empty stomach with boiled and cooled cow's milk mixed with *miśrī* (special type of sugar having big crystals).

Indications

It is an excellent recipe for promoting digestion, metabolism and positive health as well as longevity. It promotes complexion of the body. It is an effective sex tonic. Along with different types of *anupānas* or vehicles, it is used in the treatment of several obstinate and otherwise incurable diseases.

There are several variations of this recipe known as *Siddha makara dhvaja, Candrodaya makara dhvaja, Makara dhvaja vaṭī*, etc.

ACTION OF MERCURIAL PREPARATIONS

Before we move on to the next chapter, it is necessary to examine in brief the mode of action of these mercurial preparations. Mercury in the form of chloride salt, namely, Mercuric chloride and Mercurous chloride is readily absorbed from the intestine, and therefore, they produce toxic effects on the body if used continuously for a long time. While administering these preparations, special precautions are to be taken and the patient is to be given salt-free diet.

These compounds belong to the category of *nirgandha mūrcchana*, described earlier. Compounds which are discussed in this chapter—all of them contain mercury and sulphur in different proportions and their methods of preparation vary. In some of these compounds, a few other items, herbal and metallic are added during the process of preparpation. But the ultimate product remains a compound of primarily mercury and sulphur, excepting traces of other elements. Some of these additional drugs, even though added during processing, do not enter into the composition of the compound in the same proportion.

For example, during the preparation of *Rasa sindūra* and *Makara dhvaja*, with the quantum of heat applied, only mercury and sulphur could vapourise and get sublimed at the neck of the bottle. The possibility of traces of gold, etc., which are added, accompanying mercury and sulphur cannot, of course, be ruled out and these trace elements exerting considerable influence in the reticulo-endothelial system of the body, when administered internally, is a fair probability.

Even though mercury and sulphur compounds are inert, in the state of fine sub-division (which is attained by making a fine powder through continuous trituration in a mortar and pestle by adding other drugs), it gets absorbed through the mucous membrane of the intestine. While getting absorbed, these mercurial compounds affect the secretions of glandular structure lining the intestines.

This modified secretion exerts direct as well as indirect influence upon the metabolism of the person by regulating the activities of the liver, kidney and several other organs of the body. These finely sub-divided preparations of mercury and sulphur modify or inhibit the growth and virulence of the intestinal flora. These compounds also help in the growth and multiplication of the intestinal flora (saprophytes) which are useful for the body. It has been clinically observed that these mercury and sulphur compounds, even if used for considerably long time, do not produce any toxic effects like salivation and foul breath.

CHAPTER VI

PROCESSING OTHER METALS AND MINERALS

HIṄGULA (CINNABAR)

Synonyms

Hiṅgola, hiṅgula, iṅgula, mleccha, rakta, suraṅga, citrāṅga, cūrṇa pārada, rasodbhava, rañjana, kapi śīrṣaka, rakta kāya, haṃsa pāda and *darada.*

Hiṅgula is a compound of mercury and sulphur. It is pinkish red in colour and on its broken surface, white lines of mercury are found. It is naturally available in mines. But, mostly artificially prepared *hiṅgula* is available in the market and used in medicine. *Hiṅgula*, after purification, is used as such in medicinal recipes. It is also used for extraction of mercury. For both these purposes, purification of cinnabar is essential.

Adverse Effects of Impure Hiṅgula

Hiṅgula, if used without proper purification, may cause fainting, obstinate urinary disorders including stone in kidney, giddiness, blindness and fatigue.

Method of Purification

Hiṅgula should be impregnated and triturated by adding lemon juice for seven days. At the end of every day, the mortar containing *hiṅgula* should be filled up with lemon juice and kept over night before starting the process of trituration next day. Every day trituration should be done continuously for at least eight hours. After the seventh day of trituration the processed *hiṅgula* should be left in the mortar to dry up. Then it should be scrapped with the help of a knife and kept in a clean and dry glass bottle.

Properties

It alleviates all the three *doṣas* and stimulates the power of digestion. It rejuvenates the body cells and is aphrodisiac.

Indications

It is useful in the treatment of rheumatism, fever and chronic rhinitis.

Extraction of Mercury from Hiṅgula

Mercury is extracted from *hiṅgula* either by sublimation or by distillation with the help of *Ūrdhva pātana yantra* or *Tiryak pātana yantra*. This mercury should be further processed and purified before using in recipes. At least the first eight *saṃskāras*, described earlier should be performed with a view to make it absolutely free from toxicity and also for making it therapeutically more effective.

Dose

25 to 50 mg. twice daily. (*Hiṅgula* is rarely used alone).

Anupāna or Vehicle

Honey.

GANDHAKA (SULPHUR)

Synonyms

Gandha pāṣāṇa, gandhī, rasa gandhaka, sugandhika, gandhika, gandha saugandhika, pūti gandha, ati gandha, pāmāri, kīṭa nāśana, bali, bali vasā, kuṣṭhāri, śara bhūmija, śulvāri, navanīta, daityendra, gandha mādana, kīṭaghna and *krūra gandha.*

Adverse Effects of Impure Sulphur

Gandhaka, if used without purification, causes burning sensation in the body, giddiness and vitiation of blood. Impure sulphur reduces strength and complexion of the body.

Method of Purification

A stainless steel pot should be kept over an oven. Ghee, in quantity equal to that of sulphur, should be kept in it. Because of the heat, ghee will gradually melt. To this, the powder of sulphur should be added and cooked with mild fire by which the sulphur will gradually melt.

In another stainless steel pot, cow's milk should be kept upto 2/3rd of its capacity. A thin and clean cloth should be tied to its brim. The melted sulphur kept in the first pot should be gradually poured into the second pot through the cloth. When it will come into contact with the milk kept inside the pot, the sulphur will solidify. It should then be removed from the milk, washed with warm water and dried. This process should at least be repeated for three times. Every time, fresh milk should be used and milk used earlier should be thrown away. The dried sulphur should then be made to a fine powder and stored in a glass bottle for future use. If this process is repeated for one hundred times, then the sulphur will become absolutely clean and free from its characteristic smell.

Sulphur is used both externally and internally either alone or in combination with other drugs. It is used externally in the form of ointment, etc. For external use, purification of sulphur is not essential. But internally, it should never be used without purification irrespective of its use alone or in combination with other drugs.

Properties

Sulphur is pungent in taste, hot in potency and sweet in *vipāka* (the taste that emerges after digestion and during the process of metabolism). It is a rejuvenating agent. It is *yoga vāhin* (which enhances the properties of drugs to which it is added). It is carminative, stimulant of digestion and aphrodisiac. It alleviates *kapha* and *vāyu.*

Indications

Gandhaka alone is used in small doses in the treatment of various types of skin diseases, viz., scabies and eczema. In combination with other drugs and with different vehicles, it is useful in the treatment of consumption, bronchitis, asthma, tuberculosis and cervical adenitis.

For the purpose of rejuvenation, sulphur is used in a gradually increased dose (*Kalpa* therapy). Details of such therapies may be seen in any standard book on *Rasa śāstra.*

Dose

125 to 250 mg. twice daily.

Anupāna or Vehicle

Honey, milk or ghee.

Regimens

Sulphur is hot in potency for which while using this drug the patient should avoid heat producing diet and drinks and refrain from excessive exposure to heat.

SVARṆA (GOLD)

Synonyms

Suvarṇa, draviṇa, hiraṇya, kāñcana, hema, agni bīja, kanaka, jāmbū nada, jāta rūpa, rukma, cāmī kara and *hāṭaka.*

This metal in its pure form is reddish yellow in colour. Gold, which is free from chemical impurities should be used in medicine after purification.

Adverse Effects of Impure Gold

Gold, if used without proper purification may reduce the strength and intellect of individual.

Method of Purification

The leaves of gold should be taken in forceps and made red hot by exposing to the strong flame of fire. Then it should be immersed in til oil. When it becomes cold it should be taken out of it and again heated over the flame of fire. Thereafter, it should be immersed in til oil again. This process should be performed for seven times in total. In the same way, these gold leaves should be heated and immersed for seven times in each of butter-milk, cow's urine, *kāñjī* (a type of vinegar) and the decoction of *kulattha* (*Dolichos biflorus* Linn.). At the end, these leaves should be washed with warm water, dried and used for n[illegible]a.

Māraṇa

Metals like gold, etc., are therapeutically used only in the form of *bhasma*. By this process, gold becomes free from toxicity and gets easily absorbed into the body through the intestinal canal. This process also helps in increasing the therapeutic efficacy of the drug.

Purified gold is added with equal quantity of *malla* (arsenic) and triturated in a mortar and pestle by adding the juice or decoction of *kāñcanāra* (*Bauhinia variegata* Linn.) for seven days. For another seven days, it should be triturated by adding the juice of *tulasī* (*Ocimum sanctum* Linn.). Thereafter, small and round cakes flat in shape (about one inch in diameter) should be made out of this paste and dried in sun.

These cakes are to be kept inside two earthen plates and their joint should be sealed by wrapping with seven layers of mud smeared cloth. It is called *śarāva saṃpuṭa* (see Appendix II). It should then be dried in sun and cooked in *laghu puṭa* (see Appendix II) by covering it with cow-dung cakes and igniting. When it becomes cold of its own (*svāṅga sīta*), these earthen plates should be removed from the ash of cow-dung cakes and the seal should be broken carefully. Cakes collected from inside these earthen plates are placed in a mortar. To this, 1/4th in quantity of *malla* (arsenic) is added again and it should be triturated by adding the juice or decoction of *kāñcanāra* and *tulasī* for seven days each. This process should be repeated for eight times more. In subsequent cooking *(puṭas)*, the number of cow-dung cakes should be gradually increased. At the end of ten *puṭas*, the *bhasma* or calcined powder of gold becomes pink in colour. It is then stored in a clean and dry glass bottle.

Use of Thin Gold Leaves

Some physicians use very thin leaves of gold in the place of its *bhasma* in medicine. Generally, these gold leaves, added to recipes are so thin that their absorption from the intestinal tract does not pose any problem and they are therapeutically effective into some extent. But to get the best therapeutic efficacy in a small dose and to make it absolutely free from any toxic effects, gold should be used after proper *śodhana* (purification) and *māraṇa* (calcination). If these fine leaves of gold are to be used in medicine, then these should be purified, and thereafter, adequately triturated so that the recipe becomes absolutely free from the glazed particles of this metal.

Testing of Bhasma

Some amount of gold *bhasma* should be sprinkled over water. If properly prepared, particles of this *bhasma* will not go down i.e. these particles will remain floating over the surface of water. This method of testing *bhasma* is called *vāritaratva* (floating in water). A small quantity of gold *bhasma* should be rubbed with the help of two fingers. If properly prepared, these particles will enter into the crevices of the finger tips and there will be no hard and coarse particles left. This type of testing is called *rekhā pūraṇatva* (filling the crevices of fingers). The third type of testing is to expose gold *bhasma* to strong fire added with drugs collectively called *mitra pañcaka*, viz., ghee, *guñjā* (*Abrus precatorius* Linn.), honey, borax and *guggulu* (*Commiphora mukul* Engl.). These drugs reduce the melting point of any metal, and in ordinary conditions, the metal should come back to its original form by the application of heat. But if the *bhasma* is properly prepared, then in spite of strong heat, it will remain unchanged. This type of testing is called *apunarbhavatva* (non-revivability). These methods are equally good for testing the *bhasma* of other metals also.

Properties

The *bhasma* of gold is sweet in taste and *vipāka* (taste that emerges after digestion and during metabolism). It is aphrodisiac, cardiac tonic, promoter of eye-sight as well as intellect and rejuvenating. It counteracts the toxic poisons. It promotes the complexion of the skin.

Indications

It promotes longevity, maintains youth and memory. It cures serious types of fever, particularly chronic fever, nervous disorders, heart disease, tuberculosis, afflictions of voice, chizophrenia, epilepsy, hysteria, orchitis, bronchitis, asthma, chronic diarrhoea, sprue, serious types of anemia and cancer.

Dose

10 to 25 mg. twice daily.

Anupāna or Vehicle

Butter, cream, milk or ghee. In different disease conditions, it is used along with different types of *anupānas*.

RAUPYA (SILVER)

Synonyms

Rucira, tāra, saudha, śubhraka, candra lauha, candra hāsa, rūpyaka, candra and all the Sanskrit synonyms of the moon.

Silver is white and lusturous metal. It is exceedingly maleable inasmuch as thin leaves of 1/10,000 inch thickness and very fine wire could be made out of it. It does not rust even if kept exposed to air for a long time. It is of three types, viz., (1) *sahaja* (naturally available silver from mines), (2) *khanija* (extracted from ores), and (3) *kṛtrima* (artificially prepared from base metals with the help of processed mercury). For purification and *māraṇa*, only pure natural silver or silver extracted from ores should be used and it should be made to thin leaves before processing.

Adverse Effects of Impure Silver

Use of impure silver causes burning sensation in the body, reduces vitality and metabolic process and causes constipation as well as prostration.

Purification

Silver, like gold should be purified by *nirvāpana* (heating over flame of fire and then immersing in liquids) for seven times in each of til oil, butter-milk, cow's urine, *kāñjī* (a type of vinegar) and the decoction of *kulattha (Dolichos biflorus* Linn.). Thereafter, silver leaves should be heated and immersed in the juice of the leaves of *agastya* (*Sesbania grandiflora* Pers.). This process should be repeated for three times.

Māraṇa

Purified leaves of silver should be cut into pieces with a pair of scissors, mixed with equal quantity of purified mercury and made into a fine amalgam. This should be added with equal quantity of each of purified sulphur and purified orpiment. This should be triturated for one day by adding the juice of *kumārī* (*Aloe barbadensis* Mill.). Then small *cakrikās* (round and flat cakes) of about one inch diameter should be made out of this paste and dried in the sun. These are to be kept in *śarāva sampuṭa* (two earthen plates), the joint of this should be sealed by seven layers of mud smeared cloth and dried in the sun. This should then be cooked in *laghu puṭa* (see App. II). This process should be repeated for seven times. Thereafter, it should be triturated in a mortar and pestle for one hour and kept in a dry and clean glass bottle. The colour of the *bhasma*, thus obtained, will be black. There are other methods by which one can also prepare pink coloured *bhasma*.

Properties

Silver *bhasma* is cooling, astringent and sour in taste, sweet in *vipāka* (taste that emerges after digestion and during metabolism) and laxative. It arrests the process of aging. It is unctuous, depleting and alleviator of *vāta* as well as *kapha*. It promotes vitality, strength and appetite.

Indications

It cures cardiac ailments, giddiness, insanity and seminal debility.

Dose

125 mg. of the *bhasma* twice daily.

Anupāna or Vehicle

Honey or cow's milk.

Use of Silver Leaves

Some physicians use very fine silver leaves directly in medicine. But it is always advisable to use these leaves after proper purification and *māraṇa* to get its best therapeutic effects and to make it absolutely non-toxic.

TĀMRA (COPPER)

Synonyms

Śulva, raktaka, mleccha, vaktraka, nepālīya, tryambaka, sūrya loha, arka and all the Sanskrit synonyms of the sun.

Copper is collected from two different sources, viz., from mineral ores like Copper pyrite and Copper sulphate, and from animals like earth-worm and pea-cock feather.

Adverse Effects of Impure Copper

Impure copper, if used internally, afflicts complexion and causes vomiting, giddiness, burning sensation, depletion of tissue elements, diarrhoea and fainting.

Purification

For purification, thin leaves of copper should be heated over the flame of fire and immersed for seven times in each of *til* oil, butter-milk, cow's urine, *kāñjī* (a type of vinegar) and the decoction of *kulattha* (*Dolichos biflorus* Linn.). Thereafter, a paste should be prepared by triturating rock-salt with the milky latex of *arka* (*Calotropis gigantea* R. Br. ex Ait.). Copper leaves should be smeared with this paste, heated over fire and then immersed into the juice of *nirguṇḍī* (*Vitex negundo* Linn.). This process should be repeated for seven times.

Māraṇa

Purified mercury and purified sulphur, each taken in quantity equal to copper, should be made to a *kajjalī* (fine black powder like collyrium) by triturating in a pestle and mortar. This fine powder should again be triturated by adding lemon juice. The paste, thus formed, should be smeared over the leaves of purified copper and dried in the sun. These leaves should be kept inside two earthen plates. The joint of these plates should be sealed with mud smeared cloth and dried in the sun. The *śarāva sampuṭa* or sealed earthen plates should be kept inside *gaja puṭa* (see App. II) and cooked.

After it is cooled, copper leaves should be removed from the earthen plates, added with half the quantity of sulphur and triturated by adding lemon juice. From out of this, small, round and flat cakes should be prepared, dried in the sun, kept in earthen plates as before and again cooked in *gaja puṭa.* This process should be repeated again. Thus, in three *puṭas,* copper will be reduced to *bhasma* form which is black in colour.

Amṛtī Karaṇa

Copper is strongly poisonous. If it is not properly purified and if its *bhasma* is not prepared properly, then it is likely to cause several complications like vomiting, giddiness and burning sensation. Therefore, before internal administration, it should be ensured that it is free from toxicity. As a precautionary measure, a special method is prescribed for processing the *bhasma* of copper which is called *amṛtīkaraṇa* (inculcating the effects of nectar into the *bhasma* of copper). For this purpose, copper *bhasma* should be triturated with lemon juice, made to a round bolus form and dried in the sun. The rhizome of *sūraṇa* (*Amorphophalus companulatus* Bl.) should be cut into two pieces and a hole should be made in the centre of the cut surface so as to accommodate the bolus of copper *bhasma* prepared earlier. The bolus should then be kept inside this hole and covered with other portion of *sūraṇa.* The rhizome should then be smeared with about a inch of mud and dried in the sun. This should be cooked in *gaja puṭa.* When it becomes cold of its own, then the mud should be removed by scraping with the help of a knife and the bolus of copper *bhasma* should be removed from inside the rhizome carefully. If the layer of the bolus has any greenish colour then that portion should be scrapped out through a knife and rejected. The remaining portion of the bolus should be made to a powder by triturating and kept in a glass jar.

It should then be repeatedly washed with luke-warm water till the water becomes absolutely transparent and there is no greenish or bluish colour in it whatsoever. Thereafter, the *bhasma* should be dried in the sun and stored in a clean and dry glass bottle. This process is called *amṛtī-karaṇa* and it makes the copper *bhasma* absolutely free from any toxicity.

Properties

Copper *bhasma* is bitter and astringent in taste. It is sweet in *vipāka* (taste that emerges after digestion and during metabolism) and hot in potency. It alleviates *pitta* and *kapha.*

Indications

It is useful in *jaṭhara* (obstinate abdominal diseases including ascites), anemia, piles, *kuṣṭha* (obstinate skin diseases including leprosy), bronchitis, asthma, tuberculosis, chronic rhinitis, gastritis, colic pain and oedema. It is very useful in liver disorders.

Dose

125 mg. twice daily in empty stomach. If there is nausea, it can also be given after food. It is rarely used alone. Generally, it is given in a compound form along with other drugs.

Anupāna or Vehicle

Honey is used as *anupāna* for this drug.

PITTALA (BRASS)

Synonyms

Pīta lauha, kapi lauha, āra, ārakūṭa, rīti and *rītikā.*

Pittala or brass is a mixture of copper (two parts) and zinc (one part).

Adverse Effects of Impure Brass

If the *bhasma* of brass is administered without appropriate purification and *māraṇa,* then it produces all the adverse effects of impure copper described before.

Purification

General method of purification followed for gold should also be adopted in the case of brass. That is, thin leaves of brass should be heated over flame and immersed for seven times into each of sesame oil, butter-milk, cow's urine, *kāñjī* (vinegar) and the decoction of *kulattha* (*Dolichos biflorus* Linn.). In addition to the above, brass leaves should be heated over the flame and immersed in the juice of *nirguṇḍī* (*Vitex negundo* Linn.) mixed with the powder of *haridrā* (turmeric). The process should be repeated for at least five times.

Māraṇa

The method described for the *māraṇa* of copper should be adopted also for brass.

Properties

Brass is bitter in taste, ununctuous, hot in potency and depleting of tissues.

Indications

It is useful in the treatment of *rakta pitta* (a condition characterised by bleeding from various parts of the body), *kṛmi* (parasitic infestation), *kuṣṭha* (obstinate skin diseases including leprosy) and serious types of anemia.

Dose

125 mg. twice daily in empty stomach.

Anupāna or Vehicle

Honey.

KĀṂSYA (BELL METAL)

Synonyms

Kaṃsīya, kāṃsyaka, ghoṣa puṣpa, ghoṣaka, vahni loha and *ghoṣa.*

Bell metal is prepared by mixing four parts of copper and one part of tin.

Adverse Effects of Impure Kāṃsya

If bell metal is used without proper purification and *māraṇa,* then it will produce toxic effects described in respect of impure copper.

Purification

Thin leaves of bell metal should be heated and immersed for seven times into each of sesame oil, butter-milk, cow's urine, *kāñjī* (vinegar) and the decoction of *kulattha* (*Dolichos biflorus* Linn.). Thereafter, the leaves should be again heated and immersed in cow's urine. This process should be repeated for seven times.

Māraṇa

Purified sulphur and the purified *haratāla* (realgar), taken in quantities each equal to that of bell metal should be triturated by adding lemon juice. Purified leaves of bell metal should be smeared with this paste and made to round and flat cakes. These are to be dried in sun and kept inside two earthen plates. The joint of these plates should be sealed by seven layers of mud smeared cloth. Thereafter, the *śarāva sampuṭa* (earthen plates containing the drugs) should be dried in the sun and then cooked in *gaja puṭa*. This process should be repeated for four times more by which the bell metal is reduced to a fine powder form *(bhasma)*.

Properties

Bell metal is light, bitter in taste, hot in potency, depleting of tissues and promoter of eye-sight.

Indications

The *bhasma* of bell metal is useful in the treatment of *kṛmi* (parasitic infestation) and *kuṣṭha* (obstinate skin diseases including leprosy).

Dose

125 mg. twice daily.

Anupāna or Vehicle

Honey.

SVARṆA MĀKṢIKA (COPPER PYRITE)

Synonyms

Suvarṇa mākṣika, hema mākṣika, mākṣika, tāpya and *dhātu mākṣika.*

It is a compound of copper, iron and sulphur. In appearance it looks yellow like gold. Ancient ayurvedic works describe the presence of gold particles in this metallic ore. A variety of *mākṣika* containing more of iron is called *raupya mākṣika* (Iron pyrite).

Adverse Effects of Impure Mākṣika

If copper pyrite is administered without proper purification and *māraṇa*, it causes impairment of eye-sight, suppression of the power of digestion, *kuṣṭha* (obstinate skin diseases including leprosy) and *halīmaka* (serious type of jaundice).

Purification

Three parts of copper pyrite and one part of rock-salt should be made to a powder and kept in an iron pan. To this, lime juice should be added. The iron pan should be kept over fire. The powder of copper pyrite and rock-salt should be stirred with the help of an iron spatula. The process should be continued till the ingredients become red like fire. Thereafter, the iron pan should be removed from fire and allowed to cool down. The powder should then be removed and repeatedly washed with warm water till the salt content of it is completely removed. Thus, the copper pyrite becomes purified.

Māraṇa

Three parts of purified copper pyrite and one part of purified sulphur should be triturated in a pestle and mortar by adding the juice of *kumārī* (*Aloe barbadensis* Mill.). From out of this paste, round and flat cakes should be prepared and dried in sun. This should be kept in *śarāva sampuṭa* (inside two earthen plates with their joint sealed by seven layers of mud smeared cloth) and cooked in *gaja puṭa*. This process should be repeated for ten times. At the end, the *bhasma* of copper pyrite is prepared. During the second and subsequent *puṭas* less of heat should be applied.

Properties

Copper pyrite is bitter and sweet in taste. It is cold in potency, pungent in *vipāka* (taste that emerges after digestion and during metabolism) and light. It eliminates *pitta* and *kapha*, promotes strength and is rejuvenating. It is *yoga vāhin* (which accentuates the efficacy of another drug to which it is added).

Indications

It cures tuberculosis, anemia, *kuṣṭha* (obstinate skin diseases including leprosy), *grahaṇī* (sprue syndrome), piles, jaundice and hoarseness of voice.

Dose

125 mg. twice daily.

Anupāna or Vehicle

Honey, ghee or milk.

RAUPYA MĀKṢIKA (IRON PYRITE)

The term *mākṣika* generally means *svarṇa mākṣika* (copper pyrite). It has a variety which is called *raupya mākṣika* or iron pyrite.

Purification

Raupya mākṣika should be added with 1/4th in quantity of sulphur. This should be triturated for one day in a pestle and mortar by adding lemon juice. Thereafter, it should be dried. This process is to be repeated for seven times.

Māraṇa

Iron pyrite purified in the above manner should be made to small cakes and dried in sun. These cakes have to be kept inside *śarāva sampuṭa* and cooked in *laghu puṭa*. This process has to be repeated for seven times. Before each *puṭa* (cooking), 1/4th in quantity of sulphur is to be added to the *raupya mākṣika*, and it should be triturated by adding lemon juice.

Properties & Therapeutic Indications

Raupya mākṣika has the same properties and therapeutic indications as those of *svarṇa mākṣika*. Of course, it is slightly inferior in potency.

Dose

125 to 250 mg. twice daily.

Anupāna or Vehicle

Honey.

TUTTHA (COPPER SULPHATE)

Synonyms

Tutthaka, tutthāñjana, mayūraka, sasyaka, tāmra garbha and *śīkhi grīva.*

Copper sulphate is available in nature. It is also prepared artificially. Copper sulphate is soluble in water. If there are impurities, then copper sulphate solution should be filtered with the help of a filter paper. For preparation of solution, 10 gm. of the powder of copper sulphate should be mixed with five litres of warm water. After filtering, the solution should be further boiled over mild heat. Then copper sulphate will be available in solid form.

Adverse Effects of Impure Copper Sulphate

Copper sulphate, if used without purification, will produce all the toxic effects described for impure copper.

Purification

Copper sulphate should be impregnated with the decoction of *triphalā* (*harītakī* or *Terminalia chebula* Retz., *bibhītakī* or *Terminalia belerica* Roxb. and *āmalakī* or *Emblica officinalis* Gaertn.--all taken in equal quantities). This process of impregnation and trituration should be repeated thrice.

Māraṇa

Purified copper sulphate should be dried in sun and added with ghee and honey—each taken in quantity equal to that of copper sulphate. Thereafter, small cakes should be made out of the paste, kept in *śarāva sampuṭa* and cooked in *laghu puṭa*. This process should be repeated thrice.

Properties

Tuttha is pungent and astringent in taste, hot in potency, light and laxative. It scrapes out pus, etc., from putrified ulcers. It eliminates *pitta* and *kapha* and promotes eye-sight.

Therapeutic Indications

It is useful in the treatment of poisoning, piles, *kuṣṭha* (obstinate skin diseases including leprosy), *śvitra* (leucoderma), *kṛmi* (parasitic infestations) and chronic ulcers.

Dose

Generally, copper sulphate is used externally in the form of an ointment. For internal administration, it is used in the dose of 125 mg. twice daily. As a single drug, its use is very rare.

VAṄGA (TIN)

Synonyms

Vaṅgaka, raṅga, raṅgaka, śukra lauha, kurūpya and *trapu.*

Tin is available in nature. It is also available in the form of ore from which the metal is extracted. Chemically, pure tin is white, smooth and dazzling.

Adverse Effects of Impure Tin

If tin is administered in impure form, it causes several types of diseases e.g. *gulma* (phantom tumour), *prameha* (obstinate urinary disorders including diabetes), conjunctivitis, anemia, oedema, heart diseases, fistula-in-ano and renal stone.

Purification

Tin should be heated over flame and immersed for seven times in each of the sesame oil, butter-milk, cow's urine, *kāñjī* (a type of vinegar) and decoction of *kulattha* (*Dolichos biflorus* Linn.). After this general purification, tin should be kept in an iron pan till it melts. To this, powder of turmeric should be added. In another narrow mouth jar, lime-water should be kept. The mouth of this jar should be covered with a cloth. Through this cloth, the molten tin should be poured over the lime water. When it will come in contact with the lime-water it is likely to splash and the physician who is engaged in the purification process is likely to get injured. Even the jar may get broken. Therefore, it is necessary to always use a metallic jar and the mouth of the jar should be covered with a tough cloth so that particles of tin while splashing do not come out of the jar. This process should be repeated for seven times.

Māraṇa

Purified tin should be kept in an iron pan and heated till it melts. After melting, powder of *apāmārga* (*Achyranthes aspera* Linn.), 1/4th in quantity of tin, should be poured over it in small quantities and stirred with the help of a thick iron rod or spoon. When all the powder of *apāmārga* is poured, the pan should be covered with another iron pan or earthen plate and then exposed to strong heat till the iron pan becomes red hot. After it gets cooled down, the powder should be taken out and triturated by adding the juice of *kumārī* (*Aloe barbadensis* Mill.) for one day. Cakes should be made out of the paste, dried in sun and kept inside *śarvāva sampuṭa* and cooked in *gaja puṭa*. This process should be repeated for seven times.

Properties

Generally, in *bhasma* form, tin stimulates digestive power and promotes intellect. It is cold in potency. It promotoes complexion and body vitality. By promoting metabolism it helps in increasing the tissues of the body.

Therapeutic Indications

Generally, in *bhasma* form, it is useful in the treatment of all types of *prameha* (obstinate urinary disorders including diabetes). It is specially useful in preventing premature ejaculation of semen.

Dose

125 to 250 mg. twice daily.

Anupāna or Vehicle

Honey, cream of milk or fresh butter-milk.

NĀGA (LEAD)

Synonyms

Sīsaka, sīsa, nāgaka, kuvaṅgaka, kuraṅga, sindūra, kāraṇa and all the Sanskrit synonyms of *nāga* (cobra snake).

Lead is available in nature in pure form and also in the form of several chemical compounds like Lead sulphate and Lead oxide.

Adverse Effects of Impure Lead

Lead used without proper purification and *māraṇa* reduces the complexion of the body and causes *kuṣṭha* (obstinate skin diseases including leprosy), pain in joints, hemiplegia, *gulma* (phantom tumour), *prameha* (obstinate urinary disorders including diabetes), oedema, fistula-in-ano, swelling in scapular joints and colic pain.

Purification

Lead should be heated (mildly) and immersed in the juice of sesame oil, butter-milk, cow's urine, *kāñjī* (a type of vinegar) and decoction of *kulattha* (*Dolichos biflorus* Linn.) seven times in each. In addition to this general method of purification, special method of purification has to be followed to make the lead absolutely free from toxicity. In an iron spoon, lead should be heated further till it melts. To this, 1/4th in quantity of turmeric powder should be added. In another pot, juice of the leaves of *sinduvāra* (*Vitex negundo* Linn.) should be kept. This jar should be covered with an earthen plate having a hole in the centre. Through this hole, the above mentioned molten lead should be carefully poured. This process should be repeated at least for seven times. In the place of *sinduvāra* juice, lime water can also be used.

Māraṇa

In an iron pan lead should be melted. To this, the powder of the bark of *aśvattha* (*Ficus religiosa* Linn.) should be added in small quantities and rubbed with the help of a strong iron spoon till the whole lead is reduced to ash. In total, the quantity (weight) of the powder of *aśvattha* bark should be the same as that of lead. After the lead is reduced to ash, it should be collected in the centre of the iron pan and be covered with another iron plate. Thereafter, strong heat should be employed till the iron pan becomes red hot. After it cools down of its own, the powder contained in it should be washed with hot water till it becomes absolutely free from the ash of *aśvattha* (*Ficus religiosa* Linn.) bark. To the powder of lead thus obtained, equal quantity of *manaḥ śīlā* (realgar) should be added and with the juice of lemon it should be triturated for about eight hours. Thereafter, cakes should be made out of the paste, dried in sun, kept in *śarāva sampuṭa* and cooked in *laghu puṭa*. This process should be repeated for three times to make lead absolutely free from any adverse effect.

Properties

The *bhasma* of lead is sweet in taste, hot in potency, heavy, unctuous, *lekhana* (which scrapes out the tissues particularly pus, etc., from chronic ulcers), laxative, aphrodisiac and stimulant of digestion and metabolism. It alleviates *vāyu*.

Therapeutic Indications

Nāga bhasma is useful in the treatment of menorrhagia, piles and *prameha* (obstinate urinary disorders including diabetes). It is useful in the treatment of seminal debility and infection in the genito-urinary tract.

Dose

70 to 125 mg. twice daily.

Anupāna or Vehicle

Honey.

SINDŪRA (RED LEAD)

Synonyms

Giri sindūra, mahilā bhāla bhūṣaṇa, gaṇeśa bhūṣaṇa, nāgaja, nāga garbha, nāga reṇuka, māṅgalya and *bhāla saubhāgya.*

Sindūra, chemically, is a compound of lead and oxygen. It is available in nature in mines. It is also prepared artificially by heating lead in the presence of oxygen.

Sindūra or red lead is generally used externally in the form of ointment. It is only available in the form of powder. Therefore, physicians do not purify *sindūra* and use it in the form in which it is available in the market.

Properties

It is hot in potency. It is disinfectant and it helps in joining broken bones.

Therapeutic Indications

In the form of ointment, it is used in the treatment of fracture of bones, chronic ulcers, erysipelas, eczema, herps and scabies. For the preparation of ointment, ghee (preferably preserved cow's ghee) or bee's wax is used as a vehicle.

MṚDDĀRA ŚṚṄGA (LITHARGE)

Synonyms

Vodāra śṛṅgaka, mudra śaṅkha and *murdā śaṅkha.*

It is a chemical compound of lead and oxygen. It is available as such in nature from the mines. It is also artificially prepared.

Purification

Litharge should be made to a fine powder by triturating in pestle and mortar and kept in a glass container. Concentrated solution of rock salt should be added in sufficient quantity so that it remains 2" above the level of litharge powder. With the help of a piece of wood, it should be slowly stirred at least once in a day. After every seventh day, the salt solution should be replaced.

Thus, it should be kept in salt solution for at least 40 days. Thereafter, it should be washed with ordinary water at least for seven times. Then the powder should be dried and kept in a properly sealed glass bottle. It is generally used externally in the form of an ointment. Some physicians also use this powder internally in the treatment of *kṛmi* (intestinal parasitic infestation).

Properties

It is cold in potency and it alleviates *vāyu* and *kapha*.

Therapeutic Indications

It is used externally in the form of an ointment in the treatment of eczema, scabies and chronic putrified ulcers. It is specially useful in the treatment of syphilitic sores. It is also used for joining the broken bones. As a cosmetic, medicated oil prepared by boiling with litharge is used for giving black colour to the hair and beard.

SAUVĪRĀÑJANA (LEAD SULPHATE)

Añjana is of three types, namely *sauvīrāñjana* (galena or Lead sulphate), *srotoñjana* (Antimony sulphate) and *nīlāñjana* (stybnitis). There is a controversy about the identification of different types of *añjana*. Ayurvedic works written in different ages have described physical characteristics of different types of *añjana* differently. According to some, even Antimony sulphate should be taken as *sauvīrāñjana*. Accordingly, there is a mix up of synonyms of different types of *añjana*.

Synonyms

Sauvīra, suvīraja, kṛṣṇāñjana and *kālāñjana*.

Purification

Gelena should be made to a powder and impregnated with the juice of lemon, triturated and exposed to sun for eight hours. Thereafter, it should be washed with warm water, dried in sun and stored in a glass bottle. Generally, *sauvīrāñjana* is used externally as collyrium, and therefore, its *māraṇa* is not considered necessary.

Properties

It is cold in potentcy, unctuous and heavy. It is astringent in taste.

Therapeutic Indications

It is generally used in the treatement of eye-diseases including myopoeia, hypermetropoeia, cataract, conjuctivitis, glaucoma and corneal opacity. It is also used for cleaning and healing of ulcers. Internally, it is used in the treatment of *rakta-pitta* (a disease characterised by bleeding from different parts of body) and menorrhagia. If used properly, it causes menopause and thus works as an oral contraceptive.

Dose

Internally, it is used in the dose of 125 mg. twice daily.

Anupāna or Vehicle

Rice-wash *(taṇḍulodaka).*

YAŚADA (ZINC)

Synonyms

Yaśada, jaśada, rīti hetu and *kharparaja.*

It is available in the mines in the form of Zinc carbonate.

Adverse Effects of Impure Zinc

If zinc is used without proper purification and *māraṇa* it causes *gulma* (phantom tumour), *prameha* (obstinate urinary disorders including diabetes), consumption and *kuṣṭha* (obstinate skin diseases including leprosy).

Purification

Zinc should be made into small pieces, heated over flame and immersed for seven times into each—sesame oil, butter-milk, cow's urine, *kāñjī* (a type of vinegar) and the decoction of *kulattha* (*Dolichos biflorus* Linn.). After this general method, special method of purification should be followed. Zinc should be kept in an iron spoon and melted over fire. In a metal jar, cow's urine should be kept. The mouth of the jar should be covered with a plate having a hole in the centre. The melted zinc should be poured through this hole into the cow's urine. This process should be repeated for 21 times. Thereafter, zinc should be washed with warm water and dried.

Māraṇa

Zinc should be melted in an iron pan. To this, equal quantity of the powder of *bhaṅgā* (*Cannabis sativa* Linn.) and poppy pod should be poured in small quantities. While pouring this powder, zinc should be rubbed with the help of a strong iron spoon. When all the zinc gets reduced to ash, another iron plate should be kept over the pan and strong heat should be applied below till the iron pan becomes red hot. Thereafter, it should be allowed to cool of its own. It should then be washed for separating the ash of the powder added to it and dried. Then it should be triturated by adding the juice of *kumārī* (*Aloe barbadensis* Mill.). Small cakes should be made out of the paste, dried in sun and kept in *śarāva sampuṭa* and cooked in *gaja puṭa*. This process should be repeated for seven times.

Properties

The *bhasma* of zinc is astringent as well as bitter in taste and cold in potency. It alleviates both *kapha* and *pitta*.

Therapeutic Indications

It is exceedingly useful in eye-diseases for which it is used both internally and externally in the form of collyrium. It is used in the treatment of *prameha* (obstinate urinary disorders including diabetes), anemia and bronchial asthma.

Dose

125 to 250 mg. twice daily.

Anupāna or Vehicle

Honey, butter or cream of milk.

PUṢPĀÑJANA (ZINC OXIDE)

Puṣpāñjana is available in nature from the mines and is also prepared artificially by heating zinc.

It is generally used externally in the form of collyrium or ointment. Therefore, it does not require any purification or *māraṇa*.

Properties

Zinc oxide is cool in potency and unctuous.

Therapeutic Indications

It is promoter of eye-sight. It cures conjunctivitis, trachoma, eczema, scabies, chronic ulcers and burning sensation in the body (for which it is used externally as a lotion). Internally, it is used in the treatment of serious type of hic-cup.

Dose

125 to 250 mg. twice daily.

Anupāna or Vehicle

Honey and milk.

RASAKA OR KHARPARA (CALAMINE)

Synonyms

Kharparaka, yaśada kāraṇa, rīti kṛt and *tāmra rañjaka.*

It is zinc ore. It is of two types, viz. *dardura* and *kāravellaka*.

Adverse Effects of Impure Calamine

Calamine if used without proper *śodhana* and *māraṇa* will cause all the adverse effects described in respect of impure zinc.

Purification

Pieces of calamine should be heated over flame and immersed in lemon juice for seven times. Thereafter, it should be washed with hot water and dried in the sun.

Māraṇa

Purified calamine should be made to a powder and kept in pestle and mortar. To this, equal quantity of purified mercury should be added and triturated till the whole thing is reduced to a fine powder form. This powder should be kept in *śarāva sampuṭa* and cooked in *laghu puṭa*. This process should be repeated for three times.

Properties

The *bhasma* of calamine is pungent and astrigent in taste, cold in potency, light, *lekhana* (which depletes tissue elements and takes away pus, etc., from the ulcer), laxative and promoter of eye sight. It alleviates *kapha* and *pitta*.

Therapeutic Indications

It is useful in the treatment of eye-diseases, *prameha* (obstinate urinary disorders including diabetes), stone in urinary tract and *kuṣṭha* (obstinate skin diseases including leprosy). It is specially useful in the treatment of tuberculosis and chronic pyrexia.

Dose

60 to 250 mg. twice daily.

Anupāna or Vehicle

Honey.

LAUHA (IRON)

Iron is of three types, viz., *muṇḍa* or pig iron, *tīkṣṇa* or steel and *kānta* or magnetic iron.

Synonyms

Synonyms of *muṇḍa* are *muṇḍa lauha, kṛṣṇa lauha, śilātmaja, kṛṣṇāyasa, dṛṣad sāra* and *āyasa*.

Synonyms of *tīkṣṇa lauha* are *loha, lauha, lohaka, śastra lauha, tīkṣṇaka, śara lauha, kāla lauha* and *ayas*.

Synonyms of *kānta lauha* are *kānta* and *ayas kānta*.

Iron is generally extracted from the ore. For therapeutic purposes generally the *bhasma* of steel is used.

Adverse Effects of Impure Iron

If iron without proper purification and *māraṇa* is used, it causes heart disease, *kuṣṭha* (obstinate skin diseases including leprosy), colic pain, burning sensation all over the body, impotency, serious type of constipation and stone in urinary tract.

Purification

Thin leaves of iron should be heated over flame and immersed for seven times in each of sesame oil, butter-milk, cow's urine, *kāñjī* (a type of vinegar) and decoction of *kulattha* (*Dolichos biflorus* Linn.). After this general method of purification, iron should be processed again according to a special method. For this purpose, pulp of *triphalā* (see Appendix I) should be made to powder and taken in the quantity of 16 *palas* (about 750 gm.). To this, four times of water should be added, boiled and reduced to 1/4th. Then the decoction should be filtered through a cloth. Purified iron chips should be heated and immersed into this decoction for seven times. This is the special method of purification of iron.

To make iron therapeutically more effective, it is necessary to process it further. Purified iron chips should be kept inside an earthen jar. To this, sufficient quantity of cow's urine should be added to ensure that all the iron pieces are submerged. This jar should be covered with an iron plate and kept in the sun. When the cow's urine gets dried up, more cow's urine should be added to this. This process should be continued for one month. Thereafter, these iron chips are to be impregnated with the decoction of *triphalā* (see Appendix I) and the juice of *kumārī* (*Aloe barbadensis* Mill.)--for one month in each. At the end of three months, iron chips will become very fragile. This should be washed with warm water, dried and made to a powder by triturating in a pestle and mortar. This powder is to be used for *bhasma*.

Māraṇa

The above mentioned powder of iron should be impregnated and triturated with cow's urine for three days. From this paste, small cakes should be made out, kept in *śarāva sumpuṭa* and cooked in *gaja puṭa*. This process should be repeated for three times. Subsequently, it is to be cooked for three times by impregnating and triturating with the decoction of *triphalā* (see Appendix I). Seventh, eighth and ninth *puṭas* should be given by impregnating and triturating with the juice of *kumārī*. Tenth, eleventh and twelfth *puṭas* should be given by impregnating and triturating with the juice of *punarnavā* (*Boerhaavia diffusa* Linn.). The 13th *puṭa* should be given by adding 1/12th of purified *hiṅgula* (cinnabar) and triturating with the latex of *arka* (*Calotropis gigantea* R. Br. ex. Ait.). While the first twelve *puṭas* are given by cooking in *gaja puṭa*, for the 13th *puṭa* only half *gaja puṭa* should be used. It has to be cooked twice more according to the process described for the 13th *puṭa*. Thus, by cooking for 15 times, iron is reduced to *bhasma* form, which is therapeutically very useful.

Svayaṃ Agni Lauha Bhasma

Bhasma of any metal, including iron, should be tested before administration to a patient. The methods of testing are already described, viz. (1) *rekhā pūraṇatva* i.e. if the *bhasma* of iron is rubbed between two fingers then the entire quantity of *bhasma* should go into the crevices of the skin of the fingers, (2) *apunarbhavatva* i.e. if the *bhasma* of iron is added with *mitra pañcaka* (see Appendix I) and strongly heated, then it should not go back to its original metallic form, and (3) *vāri taratva* i.e. if a small quantity of iron *bhasma* is sprinkled over the surface of water, then it should float. In the case of iron, it is difficult to satisfy the 3rd test i.e. *vāri taratva*. For this purpose, the *bhasma* has to be specially processed which is called *Svayaṃ agni lauha bhasma*. To achieve this, one part of purified mercury and one part of purified sulphur should be triturated in a pestle and mortar and *kajjalī* (fine powder like collyrium) should be prepared. To this, equal quantity of iron *bhasma* should be added and triturated for six hours by adding the juice of *kumārī* (*Aloe barbadensis* Mill.). The paste should then be made to a round bolus form and covered with the leaves of *eraṇḍa*. To keep leaves of *eraṇḍa* (*Ricinus communis* Linn.) adhered to the bolus, it will be necessary to tie these leaves with the help of a thread. It should then be kept in a copper vessel and exposed to strong heat of sun for six hours. Thereafter, it should be covered with the help of another copper vessel and the joint of these two copper vessels should be sealed by wrapping with seven layers of mud smeared cloth. This should then be dried in the sun and kept inside a heap of corn for 3 days. Then the seal should be broken, leaves of *eraṇḍa* should be carefully removed and the bolus should be triturated in a pestle and mortar for three days. The powder, thus obtained, should be strained through a tough muslin cloth, and kept in a bottle. This *bhasma*, if sprinkled over the surface of water, will float. This is therapeutically very effective.

Properties

Lauha bhasma is sweet and bitter in taste, sweet in *vipāka* (the taste that develops after digestion), cold in potency, heavy, ununctuous and promoter of eye-sight, strength, virility, complexion and intellect. It alleviates *kapha* and *pitta*.

Therapeutic Indications

It is useful in the treatment of *pāṇḍu* (anemia), consumption, obesity, *kṛmi* (parasitic infestations) and oedema. It cures diseases of liver and spleen, bronchial asthma, chronic bronchitis, nephritis, heart diseases, leucorrhea, diabetes and nervous disorders.

Dose

125 to 200 mg.

Anupāna or Vehicle

Honey and ghee.

MAṆḌŪRA (RUST OF IRON)

Synonyms

Kiṭṭa, lauha bhava, lauha kiṭṭa, lauha mala and *lauhocchiṣṭa.*

In ancient times when iron was being extracted from iron ore, the residue also containing the mineral used to be thrown out and get rusted. This is called *maṇḍūra*. It should be minimum 50 years old. The best type of *maṇḍūra* is that which is 100 years old. Fresh *maṇḍūra* is not useful therapeutically.

Adverse Effects of Impure Maṇḍūra

Maṇḍūra, if administered without proper purification and *māraṇa*, produces the same type of adverse effects as those of impure iron.

Purification

Maṇḍūra should be made red hot over the flame of fire and immersed in cow's urine for seven times. Thereafter, with the help of hammer, it should be made to small pieces and by triturating in a pestle and mortar, it should be made to a fine powder.

Māraṇa

Maṇḍūra should be impregnated and triturated with the decoction of *triphalā* (see Appendix I). From the paste, cakes should be prepared, dried in sun, kept in *śarāva sampuṭa* and cooked in *gaja puṭa*. This process should be repeated for 30 times.

Properties

Maṇḍūra is cold in potency, stimulant of digestion as well as metabolism and alleviator of *pitta*.

Therapeutic Indications

It is exceedingly useful in the treatment of anemia and jaundice. It cures oedema, disorders of liver and spleen more effectively in comparison to the *bhasma* of iron.

Dose

1 gm. twice daily.

Anupāna or Vehicle

Honey.

KĀŚĪŚA (IRON SULPHATE)

Synonyms

Kāśīśaka, kāśīsa, puṣpa kāśīsa, pāṃśuka, pāṃśu kāśīsa and all Sanskrit synonyms of *khaga* (bird).

Iron sulphate is available naturally, and it is also prepared artificially. *Kāśīsa* is of two types. A variety of it is called *vimala*. Chemically, both *kāśīsa* and *vimala* are Iron sulphate.

Adverse Effects of Impure Kāśīsa

Kāśīsa, administered without proper purification and *māraṇa* produces all adverse effects described in respect of impure iron.

Purification

Kāśīsa should be made into small pieces and impregnated as well as triturated with the juice of *bhṛṅga rāja* (*Eclipta alba* Hassk.) for three days consecutively. Thereafter, it should be dried.

Mārana

Purified Iron sulphate should be treated by adding lemon juice and small cakes should be made out of it. These cakes should be dried in the sun and kept in *śarāva samputa*. This *śarāva samputa* should be cooked in *varāha puṭa* (see Appendix II). This process should be repeated till it becomes free from sour taste. Normally, seven *puṭas* are required for appropriate *māraṇa* of Iron sulphate.

Properties

Kāśīsa is sour and astringent in taste. It is hot in potency. It transforms grey hair into black and promotes strength as well as eye-sight.

Therapeutic Indications

It is useful in the treatment of leucoderma, serious type of anemia and splenic disorders. It is emenagogue. It is used externally in the form of an ointment or medicated oil for the treatment of prolapse rectum and uterus.

Dose

125 to 250 mg. twice daily in empty stomach.

Anupāna or Vehicle

Powder of *triphalā* (see Appendix I) and honey.

GAIRIKA (RED OCHRE)

Synonyms

Gairika, giri mṛt, giri mṛttikā, rakta dhātu, lauha dhātu and *giri mṛdbhava.*

It is an iron ore. It is of two types, viz. *pāṣāṇa gairika* and *svarṇa gairika*. The former is hard and the latter is soft to touch. The former is generally used for painting, etc., and the latter is preferably used in medicine.

Adverse Effects of Impure Gairika

Gairika used in impure form causes all adverse effects described in respect of impure iron.

Purification

Red ochre should be made to a powder and impregnated as well as triturated with cow's milk for three days. Red ochre is used only in purified form and its *māraṇa* is not necessary.

Properties

Red ochre is sweet and astringent in taste, cold in potency and unctuous. It promotes eye-sight.

Therapeutic Indications

It is useful in the treatment of skin diseases like itching, erysipelas, burn, scalds, piles, *rakta pitta* (a disease characterised by bleeding from different parts of the body), vomiting, hic-cup and burning syndrome. It is specifically useful in the treatment of urticaria.

Dose

1 to 2 gm. twice daily in empty stomach. It is used externally in the form of an ointment for skin diseases, burns and scalds.

Anupāna or Vehicle

Honey and milk.

ABHRAKA (MICA)

Synonyms

Gagana, bhṛṅga, abhra, kha, vyoma, vajra, ghana, girija, bahu patra, anantaka, ākāśa, ambara, śubhra, amala, garaja-dhvaja, megha and *antarikṣa*. Most of them are the synonyms of the sky or the cloud.

Mica is of four types, depending upon its colour, viz., white, pink, black and yellow. The white variety, which is commonly available, is called muscovite, the black variety, which is very useful for therapeutic purposes, is called biotite mica. This biotite mica is again of four types, viz., (1) *pināka*, (2) *nāga*, (3) *maṇḍūka*, and (4) *vajra*. If the biotite mica is kept over fire, and hissing sound comes out of it, then it is called *nāga*.

If the biotite mica is placed over fire and its layers swell, crack and splash (jump) like a frog then it is called *maṇḍūka*. The biotite mica which when placed over fire does not undergo any change is called *vajra* (literally thunder bolt). It is this *vajra* variety of biotite mica which should be used in medicine. All the other varieties are likely to produce adverse effects and therapeutically these are not very effective.

Adverse Effects of Impure Mica

Mica, administered without appropriate purification and *māraṇa*, causes pain in the sides of the chest, oedema, anemia and *kuṣṭha* (obstinate skin diseases including leprosy).

Purification

Mica should be heated over fire and immersed in *kāñjī* for seven times. For purification, heated sheets of mica may also be immersed in cow's urine, decoction of *triphalā* (see Appendix I) or cow's milk or juice of *bhṛṅga rāja* (*Eclipta alba* Hassk.).

Māraṇa

The powder of mica should be triturated with the juice of onion, made to small cakes, dried, kept in *śarāva sampuṭa* and cooked in half *gaja puṭa*. This process should be repeated for seven times. Thereafter, with the juice (or latex) of *vāsā* (*Adhatoḍa vasica* Nees), *nirguṇḍī* (*Vitex negundo* Linn.), *ārdraka* (*Zingiber officinale* Rosc.), *guḍūcī* (*Tinospora cordifolia* Miers), *arka* (*Calotropis gigantea* R. Br. ex Ait.), *snuhī* (*Euphorbia neriifolia* Linn.) and *kumārī* (*Aloe barbadensis* Mill.), it should be triturated and cooked in half *gaja puṭa* for seven times in each. At the end of this process, it should be ensured that the powder of mica has become absolutely free from glazed particles. It should satisfy all the tests prescribed for *bhasma*, viz., *vāri taratva* (floating on the surface of water), *rekhā pūraṇatva* (entering into the crevices of finger) and *apunarbhavatva* (non-revivability).

To make the *bhasma* of mica therapeutically very potent, it is necessary to cook the *bhasma* for one hundred times *(śata puṭī)* or even one thousand times *(sahasra puṭī)*. For this purpose, the juice or latex of the above mentioned drugs should be repeatedly used. There are several other drugs prescribed in ayurvedic texts on *Rasa śāstra* for this purpose. For the treatment of specific diseases, separate groups of drugs have been prescribed in ayurvedic texts which are to be used for impregnation and trituration.

Dhānyābhraka

For getting better quality of *bhasma*, mica after purification, is specifically processed. Along with 1/4th quantity of pulses, powder of mica is tied in a piece of thick woollen cloth and soaked in water for one day. Then it is rubbed with the help of both hands and squeezed while keeping the bundle in water. The powder of mica will thus come out of the woollen cloth and get deposited in water. This water is further evaporated by boiling and the powder of mica is collected. This mica is very useful for *māraṇa* and the *bhasma* prepared out of it is very effective therapeutically.

Amṛtīkaraṇa

To make mica *bhasma* absolutely free from any adverse effects and to make it therapeutically more effective it is further processed. Ten parts of mica *bhasma* should be added with 15 parts of the decoction of *triphalā* (see Appendix I) and eight parts of cow's ghee. All these should be boiled in an iron pan for three days till the ghee and decoction get dried up and well mixed with *bhasma* of mica. This powder is useful in the treatment of diseases.

Abhraka Sattva

Mica mostly contains metals like aluminium and iron. The *bhasma* of mica should be mixed with 1/4th in quantity of the powder of borax and triturated with the juice or decoction of *muśalī* (*Chlorophytum tuberosum* Baker). This should be kept in a crucible and cooked over strong fire inflammed with the help of a blower. After about three hours of strong heat, the *sattva* or essence of mica comes out of it. This metallic *sattva* is further processed and reduced to *bhasma* form. This essence of mica *(abhraka sattva)* is generally used as a *bīja* (seed) while processing mercury both for *deha siddhi* and *lauha siddhi*. It is also used therapeutically. This is an excellent rejuvenating agent and a potent aphrodisiac. It is generally used by ayurvedic physicians in the treatment of aspermia (semen without sperm).

Properties

Mica is sweet in taste, cold in potency, unctuous, promoter of complexion, strength, eye-sight, intellect, lactation, longevity, lustre of hair and the power of digestion as well as metabolism.

Therapeutic Indications

It is useful in the treatment of chronic bronchitis, bronchial asthma, anemia, tuberculosis, chronic fever, colic pain, gastritis, sprue syndrome, urticaria, giddiness, tubercular adenitis and oedema. It is an excellent drug for rejuvenation.

Dose

125 mg. twice daily in empty stomach.

Anupāna or Vehicle

Honey, milk, ghee or the juice of herbs, specifically indicated in the treatment of respective diseases.

GAURĪ PĀṢĀṆA (ARSENIC)

Synonyms

Śaṅkha viṣa, śaṅkha mūṣa, dāru mūṣa, dāru mūṣā, mallaka, phenāśma bhasma, somala, sambala and *ākhu pāṣāṇaka.*

Arsenic is well known for its toxic manifestations in the body. But by proper purification, it is used without any adverse effect in the treatment of several obstinate and otherwise incurable diseases and it becomes a rejuvenating agent. Arsenic, in pure form, is rarely available in nature. It is generally prepared artificially. The artificial arsenic, which is available in the market, is transparent in the beginning. When preserved for a long time it comes in contact with oxygen and becomes white as well as opaque.

Adverse Effects of Impure Arsenic

Administration of impure arsenic causes burning sensation in the body, trembling and pain. It causes several skin disorders, vomiting and diarrhoea. If these poisoning effects are not corrected in time, it may lead to the death of the person.

Purification

Arsenic should be tied in a piece of cloth. In a *Dolā yantra* (see Appendix II) it should be cooked for six hours by adding cow's milk or cow's ghee or the juice of *kāravella (Momordica charantia* Linn.). It is generally used after purification and its *māraṇa* is not necessary. It evaporates at a very low temperature. Therefore, exposing it to strong heat is not desirable.

Properties

Arsenic alleviates *kapha* and *vāyu.* It promotes strength and virility. When used in small doses, it rejuvenates the body.

Therapeutic Indications

It is useful in the treatment of bronchial asthma, malaria fever, anemia, enlargement of spleen, syphilis, filaria, rheumatism and *kuṣṭha* (obstinate skin diseases including leprosy).

It is strongly contra-indicated in a patient having *paittika* type of constitution or in diseases caused predominantly by *pitta.* The person using arsenic should avoid sour and pungent food as well as drinks. The person taking arsenic or its compounds should be given milk, ghee, rice and wheat in sufficient quantity to eat and drink.

Dose

Impure arsenic, if taken in dose of 125 mg., may cause death. It is therapeutically effective in a very small dose like 1 to 2 mg. only. Therefore, it is generally used in a compound form by adding other drugs, particularly those having cooling effect (to counteract its inherent heating effect).

Anupāna or Vehicle

It is generally used along with cow's ghee or cow's milk.

HARITĀLA (YELLOW ARSENIC OR ORPIMENT)

Synonyms

Tāla, tālaka, naṭa bhūṣaṇa, naṭa maṇḍana, śailūṣa bhūṣaṇa, viḍālaka, cirta gandha, piñjara, vaṃśa patraka, āla, pītanaka and *malla gandhaja.*

It is a chemical compound of arsenic and sulphur. It is of two types, viz., *patra tālaka* and *piṇḍa tālaka*. The former is composed of layers whereas the latter looks like a piece of stone. It is the former which is preferably used in medicine.

Adverse Effects of Impure Orpiment

Orpiment, if used without proper purification and *māraṇa*, may produce adverse effects as described in respect of arsenic.

Purification

Patra tālaka type of orpiment should be made into small pieces, tied in a *poṭṭalī* (into a bolus form) with the help of a piece of cloth and cooked in *Dolā yantra* (see Appendix II) for three hours by adding *cūrṇodaka* (lime water). Thereafter, it should be again cooked in the same *Dolā yantra* for three hours by adding the juice of *kuṣmāṇḍa* (*Benincasa hispida* Cogn.), sesame oil and decoction of *triphalā* (see Appendix I) one after the other. Thereafter, pieces of yellow arsenic should be well washed with warm water, dried in the sun and made to powder.

Rasa Māṇikya

After purification, a small quantity of the powder of yellow arsenic should be kept between two sheets of mica. These two mica sheets containing yellow arsenic should be carefully taken by forceps and kept over red hot charcoal. The charcoal should be further inflammed with the help of a blower. The yellow arsenic will slowly melt and become red like ruby inside the sheets of mica. Then it should be removed from fire, and after it is cooled of its own, mica sheets should be carefully separated and the red scale like substance should be collected. This has to be triturated in a pestle and mortar, made to a fine powder and stored in a glass bottle. Generally, this process is considered as *māraṇa* of yellow arsenic and it is in this form that this drug is used in the treatment of diseases.

Properties

It is hot in potency.

Therapeutic Indications

It is used in the treatment of chronic bronchitis caused by *kapha* and *vāyu*, bronchial asthma, chronic urticaria, chronic fever, syphilis, gout, sinusitis, fistula and *kuṣṭha* (obstinate skin diseases including leprosy).

Dose

20 mg. twice daily in empty stomach.

Anupāna or Vehicle

Honey and ghee.

All dietetic restrictions mentioned for arsenic should also be followed while administering yellow arsenic.

MANAḤ ŚILĀ (Red Arsenic or Realgar)

Synonyms

Roga śilā, śilā, naipālikā, manoguptā, manojñā, nāga jihvika, kunaṭī, kulaṭī, golā, ṇāga mātā, kalyāṇikā and *rasa netrikā.*

Like orpiment, realgar is also a compound of arsenic and sulphur. But the former is yellow whereas the latter is pinkish red in colour.

Adverse Effects of Impure Realgar

If used without appropriate purification, it produces all the adverse effects described in respect of arsenic. In addition, it makes the person considerably weak and causes serious type of constipation. It also causes obstruction to micturation or painful micturation.

Purification

Manaḥ śilā should be impregnated and triturated with the juice of either *agastya* leaf (*Sesbania grandiflora* Pers.), *śṛṅgavera* (ginger), *mātuluṅga* (lemon) or *bhṛṅga rāja* (*Eclipta alba* Hassk.) for seven days. Thereafter, *manaḥ śilā* should be dried, made to powder and stored in a glass bottle. Realgar is used after purification and its *māraṇa* is not necessary.

Properties

Realgar is pungent and bitter in taste, hot in potency and rejuvenating.

Therapeutic Indications

It cures chronic bronchitis, chronic fever, bronchial asthma, itching and anemia.

Dose

20 mg. twice daily in empty stomach.

Anupāna or Vehicle

Honey or ghee.

All the dietetic restrictions, prescribed for arsenic are to be followed while administering preparation of realgar to a patient.

GODANTĪ (GYPSUM)

Synonyms

Go dantikā, go danta and *go dantā.*

It is a compound of calcium and sulphur. It is also called *godantī haritāla.* This often causes confusion to a novice who may consider it to be an arsenic compound.

Purification

Calcium sulphate should be washed with adequate quantity of warm water by which it becomes purified.

Māraṇa

Powder of purified *godantī* should be triturated by adding the juice of *kumārī* (*Aloe barbadensis* Mill.) for one day, cakes should be made out of this paste, dried in sun, kept in *śarāva sampuṭa* and cooked in *gaja puṭa* (see Appendix II). This process should be repeated for three times.

Properties

It is cold in potency and it alleviates *pitta.*

Therapeutic Indications

It is useful in the treatment of *paittika* type of fever, chronic fever, headache including migraine, anemia, tuberculosis and leucorrhea. It is also useful in chronic bronchitis and asthma. It is specially useful in the treatment of rickets in children.

Dose

1 gm. twice daily.

Anupāna or Vehicle

Honey or milk.

BADARA PĀṢĀṆA (SILICATE OF LIME)

Synonyms

Hazrul yahūda, saṅge yahūda, aśmabhid and *badarāśma.*
It is a compound of calcium and silica.

Purification

Badara pāṣāṇa is available in the market in the form of ecliptical stones of the size of *ber* fruit. It should be washed with warm water, cleaned through a cloth and dried.

Māraṇa

Badara pāṣāṇa is generally used in the form of *piṣṭī*. It does not involve application of heat or fire, made to powder simply in pestle and mortar and triturated by adding rose water or sandalwood oil for about three hours till it is reduced to a very fine powder form.

Properties

It is cold in potency. It alleviates *pitta* and is a diuretic.

Therapeutic Indications

It is used in the treatment of stone in urinary tract, dysuria and anuria.

Dose

Half to 1 gm.

Anupāna or Vehicle

Honey, milk or rose water.

ṬAṄKAṆA (BORAX)

Synonyms

Ṭaṅka, ṭaṅga, ṭaṅgaṇa, drāvaka, raṅga, raṅgada, lauha śodhana, svarṇa śodhana and *saubhāgya.*

It is generally available in the banks of lakes containing saline water.

Purification and Māraṇa

Pieces of borax should be cleaned of physical impurities like sand, mud, stone or pieces of wood. Clean borax should be kept in an iron pan and heated. When the water of crystallisation gets evaporated, it swells and comes out in the form of fragile masses. It should be collected and made to powder and kept in clean and dry glass bottle.

Properties

It is pungent in taste, hot in potency, ununctuous, laxative and expectorant.

Therapeutic Indications

It is useful in the treatment of amenorrhea, nervous disorders, chronic fever, chronic bronchitis and asthma. It causes contraction of uterus. Therefore, it is used in the event of retention of foetus in the uterus and delayed delivery. It stops bleeding from different parts of the body. Externally, it is used as an ointment in the treatment of chronic ulcer and itching in soft and tender parts of body.

Dose

125 mg. twice daily in empty stomach.

Anupāna or Vehicle

Honey.

SPHAṬIKĀ (ALUM)

Synonyms

Surāṣṭrajā, saurāṣṭrī, saurāṣṭra mṛttikā, sphuṭi, sphuṭikā, phaṭikā, śubhrā, kāṅkṣī, tuvarī, raṅgadā, dṛḍha raṅgadā and *raṅga dṛḍhā.*

Purification and Māraṇa

Alum has to be cleaned of its physical impurities like mud, sand and pieces of wood. In an iron pan, purified alum should be kept and heated. When the water of crystallisation evaporates, it will swell and become opaque as well as white. This has to be collected, made to powder and kept in a clean and dry glass bottle.

Properties

It is sweet, slightly sour and astringent in taste. It is hot in potency.

Therapeutic Indications

It is useful in the treatment of leucoderma, bleeding from different parts of the body, stomatitis and malaria fever. It is very useful for gums and teeth. It is specially used in the treatment of bleeding gums, prolapse of rectum and prolapse of uterus. It is externally used in the form of ointment and as lotions for the treatment of bleeding, ulcer, scabies and erysipelas.

Dose

250 mg. to 500 mg. three to four times per day.

Anupāna or Vehicle

Honey.

CHAPTER VII

GEMS AND JEWELS

HĪRAKA (DIAMOND)

Synonyms

Vajra, hīrā, abhedya, bhidura, kuliśa, vajraka and *bhārgava priya.*

It is one of the important jewels, and therefore, well known. Astrologically, it is used in a ring or necklace to propitiate the planet Venus. For that purpose, the physical characteristics of diamond, viz., its size, shape and transparency are described in ayurvedic and astrological texts in detail. For the purpose of medicine, these specifications are not essential and even raw and unpolished diamond can be used. It should, however, be natural diamond. Synthetic diamonds are not useful for medicinal purposes.

It is the hardest substance. Therefore, preparing *bhasma* out of it involves some special technique.

Adverse Effects of Impure Diamond

If used without proper purification and *māraṇa,* diamond may cause excruciating pain in the sides of the chest, *kuṣṭha* (obstinate skin diseases including leprosy), burning sensation all over the body and giddiness.

Purification

Pieces of diamond should be taken with forceps, heated over the flame of fire and immersed in the latex of *snuhī* (*Euphorbia neriifolia* Linn.). This process should be repeated for one hundred times. Similarly, heated pieces of diamond should be immersed in the decoction of *kulattha* for 100 times. For this purpose, it is to be heated over a strong flame of fire so that it becomes red hot like a piece of ignited charcoal. Thereafter, it should be immersed in the latex and decoction described above. Since it may not be convenient to hold the piece of diamond for such a long time with forceps, in practice, it is generally kept in a crucible *(mūṣā)* which is heated over strong fire, and from out of this crucible, the red hot diamond should be immersed into the latex and the decoction. This process serves two purposes. It makes diamond free from any toxicity and it also makes the piece of diamond very fragile so that its *māraṇa* (reducing into a fine powder form) becomes easy. After purification, diamond should be kept in a pestle and mortar and triturated. It should then be strained through a fine cloth and kept in a glass bottle.

Māraṇa

Purified fine powder of diamond should be added with equal quantity of each of *Rasa sindūra*, purified realgar, purified orpiment and purified sulphur and kept in an iron pestle and mortar. To this, the decoction of *kulattha* (*Dolichos biflorus* Linn.) should be added and triturated for three days. The paste of this should be made to a cake form, dried in sun, kept in *śarāva samputa* and cooked in *gaja puṭa*. This process should be repeated for 14 times.

Properties

Diamond, in *bhasma* form, is an excellent rejuvenating agent and *yogavāhin* (which enhances the property of another drug when added).

Therapeutic Indications

It is an excellent drug for treatment of different types of cancer, tumour, *prameha* (obstinate urinary disorders including diabetes), anemia, oedema, *udara* (obstinate abdominal diseases including ascites) and serious type of impotency. It promotes eye-sight, strength, complexion, virility and intellect.

Dose

3 to 6 mg. twice daily in empty stomach.

Since it is used in a very small quantity, it is generally mixed with other medicines like *Rasa sindūra* (about 30 times) and then administered to the patient. Depending upon the nature of the diseases, other suitable drugs can also be added to the *bhasma* of diamond and administered to the patient in a compound form.

Anupāna or Vehicle

Honey, milk, cream, sugar or musk.

MĀṆIKYA (RUBY)

Synonyms

Raṅga māṇikya, padma rāga, ravi ratna, śoṇa ratna, kuruvinda and *lohita.*

Ruby is used astrologically to propitiate the Sun. The physical characteristics of ruby, useful for astrological purposes, are described in astrological and ayurvedic works. For the purpose of medicine, raw and unpolished ruby can also be used.

Purification

Māṇikya should be cooked in *Dola yantra* (see Appendix II) by adding lemon juice for three hours. It should then be washed with warm water and dried.

Māraṇa

Māṇikya is used both in *bhasma* and *piṣṭī* forms. *Māṇikya* should be added with equal quantity of each of purified realgar, purified orpiment and purified sulphur. In an iron pestle and mortar it should be triturated by adding lemon juice. The process of trituration should be continued for seven days. Before trituration, pieces of ruby should be made into powder by pounding in an iron container. After trituration, small cakes should be made out of it, dried in sun, kept in *śarāva sampuṭa* (see Appendix II) and cooked in *gaja puṭa.* This process should be repeated for eight times. For the purpose of *piṣṭī,* raw powder or purified ruby should be triturated in an iron pestle and mortar by adding rose water. The trituration should be continued till ruby is reduced to a very fine powder form. It should then be strained through a fine cloth and stored in a glass bottle.

Properties

Ruby *bhasma* is sweet in taste, aphrodisiac, cardiac tonic and stimulant of digestion as well as metabolism.

Therapeutic Indications

It is very effective in the treatment of any type of bleeding in the body. It cures impotency and tuberculosis.

Dose

100 to 200 mg. twice daily in empty stomach.

Anupāna or Vehicle

Musk or honey.

TĀRKṢYA (EMERALD)

Synonyms

Garutmata, marakata, gāruḍa, budha ratna, rauhiṇeya and *harita ratna.*

Astrologically it is used externally to propitiate the planet Mercury.

Purification

Emerald should be cooked in a *Dolā yantra* (see Appendix II) by using cow's milk for three hours.

Māraṇa

Emerald is used both in *bhasma* and *piṣṭī* forms. The methods prescribed for ruby are to be followed for emerald also.

Therapeutic Indications

Emerald *bhasma* is useful in the treatment of chronic fever, vomiting, asthma, piles, anemia and oedema.

Dose

100 to 200 mg. twice daily in empty stomach.

Anupāna or Vehicle

Honey.

VAIDŪRYA (CAT'S EYE)

Synonyms

Vidūra ratna, ketu ratna, vidūraja, viḍālākhya, viḍālākṣa and *vāyaja.*

Astrologically this gem is used externally in a ring for propitiating the planet *Ketu* (Dragon's tail). For astrological use its appropriate physical characteristics are described in astrological and ayurvedic texts. For the purpose of medicine, raw, unpolished cat's eye is generally used.

Purification

In a *Dolā yantra,* cat's eye should be cooked for three hours by adding the decoction of *triphalā* (see Appendix I). Thereafter, it should be washed with warm water and dried.

Māraṇa

The process of *māraṇa* prescribed for ruby should be followed for cat's eye also. It should be cooked in *gaja puṭa* for eight times.

Properties

Cat's eye in *bhasma* form is sweet in taste, cooling in potency, stimulant of digestion and promoter of intellect, longevity, strength and eye-sight. It is a mild laxative.

Therapeutic Indications

Cat's eye in *bhasma* form cures *rakta pitta* (a disease characterised by bleeding from different parts of the body). It is useful in the treatment of eye diseases.

Dose

25 to 125 mg. twice daily in empty stomach.

Anupāna or Vehicle

Milk.

NĪLA (SAPPHIRE)

Synonyms

Nīlopala, nīla ratna, sunīlaka, mahā nīla, nīlāśma and *śani ratna.*

Astrologically it is used externally in a ring for propitiating the planet Saturn. Physical characteristics of sapphire that should be used for this purpose are described in astrological and ayurvedic texts.

Purification

In a *Dolā yantra,* sapphire should be cooked by adding the juice of *nīlī* (*Indigofera tinctoria* Linn.) for three hours. Thereafter, it should be washed with warm water and dried.

Māraṇa

Procedure prescribed for *māraṇa* of ruby should be followed for sapphire also.

Properties

It alleviates all the three *doṣas.* It is an aphrodisiac. It promotes digestion, metabolism, strength and complexion.

Therapeutic Indications

It is useful in the treatment of *kuṣṭha* (obstinate skin diseases including leprosy), piles, fistula-in-ano, asthma, bronchitis and malarial fever. It is very useful in the treatment of heart-diseases.

Dose

25 to 125 mg. twice daily in empty stomach.

Anupāna or Vehicle

Honey.

GOMEDA (CINNAMON STONE)

Synonyms

Gomedaka, pińga sphaṭika, rāhu ratna and *tamo maṇi.*

Astrologically it is used externally to propitiate the planet Rāhu (Dragon's head). Physical characteristics of the stone for astrological use are described in astrological and ayurvedic texts.

Purification

In a *Dolā yantra,* cinnamon stone should be cooked for three hours by adding lemon juice. Thereafter, it should be washed with warm water and dried.

Māraṇa

The procedure prescribed for the *māraṇa* of ruby should be followed for cinnamon stone also.

Properties

Cinnamon stone in *bhasma* form alleviates *kapha* and *pitta,* promotes digestion and appetite. It is hot in potency and it promotes strength.

Therapeutic Indications

It is useful in the treatment of serious types of anemia and tuberculosis.

Dose

25 to 125 mg. twice daily in empty stomach.

Anupāna or Vehicle

Milk.

VAIKRĀNTA (TOURMALINE)

Synonyms

Vikrānta, jīrṇa vajraka, kuvajra, kṣudra kuliśa and *cūrṇa vajra.*

Purification

Tourmaline should be cooked in *Dolā yantra* for three hours by adding the decoction of *kulattha* (*Dolichos biflorus* Linn.).

Māraṇa

Tourmaline should be added with equal quantity of purified sulphur and triturated by adding lemon juice. Cakes should be made out of this paste, dried in sun, kept in *śarāva samputa* and cooked in *gaja puṭa.* This process should be repeated for eight times.

Properties

Tourmaline has all the six tastes. It alleviates all the three *doṣas.*

Therapeutic Indications

It is used in the treatment of anemia, *udara* (obstinate abdominal diseases including ascites), asthma, bronchitis, tuberculosis and *prameha* (obstinate urinary disorders including diabetes).

Dose

125 to 250 mg. twice daily in empty stomach.

Anupāna or Vehicle

Honey or fresh milk.

RĀJĀVARTA (LAPIS-LAZULI)

Synonyms

Nṛpāvarta, āvarta maṇi, nṛpopala and *nīlāśma.*

Purification

Lapis-lazuli should be cooked in a *Dolā yantra* by adding lemon juice for three hours. This process should be repeated for three times.

Māraṇa

Lapis-lazuli should be added with equal quantity of purified sulphur and triturated in pestle and mortar by adding the juice of *bhṛṅga rāja* (*Eclipta alba* Hassk.). Then it should be made to cakes, dried in sun, kept in *śarāva sampuṭa* and cooked in half *gaja puṭa*. This process should be repeated for seven times.

Properties

Bhasma of lapis-lazuli is pungent and bitter in taste, cold in potency and stimulant of digestion. It is an excellent drug for rejuvenation.

Therapeutic Indications

It is useful in the treatment of asthma, *prameha* (obstinate urinary disorders including diabetes), tuberculosis and serious type of vomiting as well as hic-cup.

Dose

125 to 250 mg. twice daily in empty stomach.

Anupāna or Vehicle

Milk or fresh butter.

SAṄGE YAŚADA (ZADE)

Purification

In a *Dolā yantra*, zade is cooked by adding lemon juice for three hours. Thereafter, zade should be washed with warm water and dried.

Māraṇa

Zade is generally used in the form of *piṣṭī*. For this purpose, it is triturated by adding rose water till it is reduced to a very fine powder form which takes about ten days.

Properties

It is cold in potency.

Therapeutic Indications

It is useful in the treatment of heart diseases, colic pain, burning micturation and stone in urinary tract.

Dose

250 to 500 mg. twice daily in empty stomach.

Anupāna or Vehicle

Milk or fresh butter.

AKĪKA (AGATE)

Purification and Māraṇa

Agate should be cooked for three hours in a *Dolā yantra* by adding lemon juice. Thereafter, it should be washed, dried, made to small pieces and used for *bhasma* or *piṣṭī*. The procedure in this connection prescribed for ruby should also be adopted for agate.

Properties

It is cold in potency, ununctuous and aphrodisiac.

Therapeutic Indications

It is useful in the treatment of *rakta pitta* (a disease characterised by bleeding from different parts of the body) and diseases of the heart, gum as well as teeth. It is also useful in the treatment of stone in the urinary tract.

Dose

250 to 500 mg. twice in empty stomach.

Anupāna or Vehicle

Milk, cream or fresh butter.

SPHAṬIKA (ROCK-CRYSTAL)

Synonyms

Śiva ratna, kāca maṇi, sphaṭikāśma, sphaṭikopala, śāli piṣṭa, dhauta śāli and *amala maṇi.*

Purification and Māraṇa

For its purification and *māraṇa,* methods prescribed for lapis-lazuli should be followed.

Properties

The *piṣṭī* of rock-crystal is sweet in taste, extremely cold in potency and promoter of strength.

Therapeutic Indications

Rock-crystal is useful in the treatment of *rakta pitta* (a disease characterised by bleeding from different parts of the body), serious type of fever (with high temperature) and burning sensation all over the body.

Dose

125 to 250 mg. twice daily in empty stomach.

Anupāna or Vehicle

Milk, cream or fresh butter.

SŪRYA KĀNTA (SUN-STONE)

Synonyms

Sūrya maṇi, sūryopala, vahni garbha and *jvalanopala.*

Purification and Māraṇa

Sun-stone does not need purification. It is to be crushed into pieces, added with equal quantity of each of purified sulphur and purified realgar and triturated in a pestle and mortar till the whole thing is reduced to a fine powder. Then it should be kept in *śarāva sampuṭa* and cooked in a half *gaja puṭa*. This process should be repeated for seven times.

Properties

It is hot in potency and rejuvenating. It alleviates *vāyu* and *kapha* and promotes intellect.

Therapeutic Indications

It is useful in the diseases caused by *vāyu* and *kapha.*

Dose

125 to 250 mg. twice a day in empty stomach.

Anupāna or Vehicle

Honey or milk.

CANDRA KĀNTA (MOON-STONE)

Synonyms

Candra maṇi, candropala, śaśī kānta and *indu kānta.*

Purification

Moon-stone does not need any purification.

Māraṇa

Moon-stone should be crushed by a hammer and reduced to powder. It should be added with equal quantities of purified realgar and purified sulphur, and triturated in a pestle and mortar by adding the juice of *kumārī (Aloe barbadensis* Mill.). From this paste, cakes should be prepared, dried in sun, kept in *śarāva sampuṭa* and cooked in half *gaja puṭa*. This process should be repeated for seven times.

Properties

Moon-stone is extremely cold in potency and unctuous. It alleviates *pitta*.

Therapeutic Indications

It is useful in the treatment of *rakta pitta* (a disease characterised by bleeding from different parts of the body), burning sensation all over the body, fever with high temperature and heart-diseases.

Dose

125 to 250 mg. twice daily in empty stomach.

Anupāna or Vehicle

Milk or fresh butter.

PEROJĀ (TORQUOISE)

Synonyms

Perojaka and *peroja*.

Purification and Māraṇa

The procedure prescribed for the purification and *māraṇa* of *rājāvarta* (Lapis-lazuli) should be followed for torquoise.

Properties

Torquoise is sweet and astringent in taste. It stimulates digestion and is cold in potency.

Therapeutic Indications

It is useful in the treatment of diseases of heart and eyes. It promotes strength and activities of brain cells.

Dose

125 to 250 mg. twice a day in empty stomach.

Anupāna or Vehicle

Milk, cream or fresh butter.

TṚṆA KĀNTA (AMBER)

Synonyms

Tṛṇa kānta maṇi and *kaharubā*.

Purification and Māraṇa

Amber does not require any purification. It is generally used in the form of *piṣṭī* (thin powder form which is prepared by trituration and without exposure to heat). For this purpose, amber should be made to powder and triturated with rose water till it is reduced to a very fine powder form.

Properties

It is sweet in taste as well as *vipāka* (the taste that emerges after digestion and during metabolism) and cold in potency.

Therapeutic Indications

It is used in the treatment of heart diseases, *rakta pitta* (a disease characterised by bleeding from different parts of the body) and gastro-intestinal disorders.

Dose

125 to 250 mg. twice a day in empty stomach.

Anupāna or Vehicle

Honey, fresh butter or milk.

CHAPTER VIII

ANIMAL PRODUCTS AND ŚILĀJATU

MUKTĀ (PEARL)

Synonyms

Muktā phala, mauktika, śuktija, sauktikeya, śaśī ratna and *śaśī priya.*

In the market, three types of pearl are available, viz., (1) artificial pearl, (2) cultured pearl, and (3) natural pearl. It is the third variety which is the most useful in medicine. If natural pearl is not available, then cultured pearl can also be used in medicine but it would be slightly less effective. Artificial pearl is not at all useful in medicine.

Pearl is used astrologically in a ring or a neck-lace to propitiate the Moon. Physical characteristics of pearl, suitable for this purpose, are described in astrological and ayurvedic works.

Purification

In a *Dolā yantra,* pearl should be cooked for three hours by adding the juice of *jayantī* (*Sesbania sesban* Merr.).

Māraṇa

It is used both in the form of *bhasma* and *piṣṭī*. For *bhasma*, purified pearl should be made to small pieces and triturated with cow's milk for six hours. From this paste, cakes should be made out, dried in the sun, kept in *śarāva sampuṭa* (see Appendix II) and cooked in *laghu puṭa*. This process should be repeated thrice.

For *piṣṭī*, purified pearl should be triturated by adding rose water till it is reduced to a fine powder form.

Properties

Pearl is sweet in taste, cold in potency, stimulant of digestion and promoter of virility, longevity, eye-sight as well as complexion.

Therapeutic Indications

It is useful in the treatment of chronic fever, *dāha* (burning syndrome), teething trouble in children, diseases of bone, tuberculosis, bronchial asthma, bronchitis and heart diseases.

Dose

25 to 50 mg. twice daily in empty stomach.

Anupāna or Vehicle

Milk, cream or fresh butter.

PRAVĀLA (CORAL)

Synonyms

Pravālaka, bhauma ratna, vidruma and *abdhi jantu viśeṣottha.*

Astrologically, coral is used in a ring or neck-lace to propitiate the planet Mars. In the market it is available in two forms, viz., stem of coral and the root of the coral. It is the stem of coral which is therapeutically very useful. The root of the coral is less effective therapeutically.

Purification

Pravāla is a sea-product and is porous. Therefore, it is likely to contain sand and foreign bodies inside. The possibility is more in the case of the root of the coral. Therefore, coral should be crushed into small pieces and its physical impurities should be removed. Then it should be washed with warm water and dried. Thereafter, in a *Dolā yantra, pravāla* should be cooked for three hours by adding the juice or decoction of *jayantī* (*Sesbania sesban* Merr.). After cooking, it should again be washed with warm water and dried.

Māraṇa

Coral is used both in *bhasma* and *piṣṭī* forms. For *bhasma*, coral should be kept in a pestle and mortar and triturated by adding the juice of *kumārī (Aloe barbadensis* Mill.). From out of the paste, cakes should be made out, dried in sun, kept in *śarāva sampuṭa* and cooked in half *gaja puṭa*. This process should be repeated for three times.

For *piṣṭī*, purified coral should be triturated in a pestle and mortar by adding rose water till it is reduced to a fine powder form.

Properties

Coral is sweet and alkaline in taste, cold in potency, digestive stimulant, carminative and promoter of eye-sight.

Therapeutic Indications

Coral is useful in the treatment of chronic fever, tuberculosis, bronchitis, *raktapitta* (a disease characterised by bleeding from different parts of the body), excessive sweating, sweating at night and diseases of bone.

Dose

125 to 500 mg. twice daily in empty stomach.

Anupāna or Vehicle

Honey, milk or fresh butter.

ŚAṄKHA (CONCH-SHELL)

Synonyms

Śaṅkhaka, kambu, trirekha, samudraja, sunāda, dīrgha nāda and *kāmboja*.

Purification

Conch-shell should be broken into pieces and washed with hot water so as to remove foreign bodies like mud and sand. Then pieces of conch-shell should be cooked in a *Dolā yantra* (see Appendix II) by adding lemon juice for twelve hours. Thereafter, these pieces are to be washed again with warm water and dried.

Māraṇa

Purified pieces of conch-shell should be kept inside *śarāva sampuṭa* (see Appendix II) and cooked in *gaja puṭa*. After this cools down of its own, the seal of the *śarāva sampuṭa* should be broken carefully and pieces of conch-shell should be removed. In a pestle and mortar, these pieces are to be triturated and reduced to a powder form. Thereafter, this powder is to be kept in *śarāva sampuṭa* again and cooked in *gaja puṭa*. After this second cooking, conch-shell powder should be removed and triturated again to a fine powder form. This should be kept in an air-tight glass bottle.

Properties

It is cold in potency. It promotes the power of digestion and strength.

Therapeutic Indications

It is useful in the treatment of indigestion, diarrhoea, sprue syndrome, gastritis, gastric ulcer and deuodenal ulcer. Externally, it is used in the form of ointment for removing pimples from the skin of the face. It is also useful in eye-diseases like cataract. For this purpose, *śaṅkha bhasma* is not used because of its corrosive action. Generally, the ordinary powder of purified conch-shell is used for this purpose. Along with other drugs, it is reduced to a fine powder form and applied externally like collyrium in the treatment of cataract and other eye-diseases.

Dose

250 mg. twice daily after food.

Anupāna or Vehicle

Hot water.

VARĀṬIKĀ (COWRIE SHELL)

Synonyms

Varāṭa, varāṭaka, varāṭī, kapardaka , kapardī, kapardikā, bāla krīḍanaka, cara and *carācara.*

Cowrie-shells are of three types depending upon their colour, viz. yellow, white and brown. For medicinal purposes, yellow type of cowrie-shell of the weight of 10 to 15 gm. each is very useful.

Purification

Cowrie-shell should be cooked in a *Dolā yantra* (see Appendix II) by adding *kāñjī* for three hours. Thereafter, cowrie-shells should be kept in *śarāva sampuṭa* and cooked in *gaja puṭa.* After it cools down of its own, cowrie-shells should be removed from *śarāva sampuṭa* and triturated in a pestle and mortar till it is reduced to a very fine powder form. This powder should be kept in a dry air-tight glass bottle.

Properties

Cowrie-shell in *bhasma* form is hot in potency and stimulant of digestion.

Therapeutic Indications

Cowrie-shell *bhasma* is useful in the treatment of indigestion, peptic ulcer and sprue syndrome. It is specially useful in the treatment of intestinal tuberculosis. It is extremely useful in the treatment of eye diseases like cataract and ear diseases like otitis media.

Dose

250 mg. twice daily after food.

Anupāna or Vehicle

Hot water.

ŚUKTI (SEA-SHELL)

Synonyms

Śuktika, muktā mātā, muktā gṛha, mahā śuktī, mauktika prasavā, muktā geha and *mauktika mandira.*

Purification

Sea-shell should be cooked in a *Dolā yantra* by adding lemon juice. Thereafter, the shell should be washed with warm water.

Māraṇa

After purification, sea-shell should be reduced to small pieces with the help of a hammer, kept in *śarāva sampuṭa* and cooked in *gaja puṭa*. After this becomes cool of its own, pieces of sea-shell should be removed from *śarāva sampuṭa* and triturated in a pestle and mortar till it is reduced to a fine powder form.

Therapeutic Indications

The *bhasma* of sea-shell is useful in the treatment of colic pain, heart diseases, asthma, stone in urinary tract, diseases of spleen and *udara roga* (obstinate abdominal diseases including ascites).

Dose

250 mg. twice daily after food.

Anupāna or Vehicle

Hot water.

SAMUDRA PHENA (CUTTLE FISH-BONE)

Synonyms

Phena, suphena, phenaka, abdhi phena, ḍinḍīra and *abdhi kapha.*

Purification

The external coating (shell) of the cuttle fish-bone should be removed carefully, and triturated in a pestle and mortar by adding lemon juice till it is reduced to a fine powder form. Generally, it is used in medicine simply after purification and its calcination ***(māraṇa)*** is not necessary.

Therapeutic Indications

It is useful in the treatment of eye diseases, ear diseases like otitis media and *kuṣṭha* (obstinate skin diseases including leprosy).

MṚGA ŚṚṄGA (DEER-HORN)

Synonyms

Eṇa śṛṅga, mṛga viṣāṇaka and *hariṇa śṛṅga.*

Purification

Pieces of dear-horn should be washed with warm water to remove impurities from its exterior.

Māraṇa

Deer-horn should be cut into small pieces with the help of a saw and put in fire till it gets completely burnt. Thereafter, these pieces should be removed, kept in a pestle and mortar and triturated by adding the latex of *arka* (*Calotropis gigantea* R. Br. ex Ait.). Small cakes should be made out of this paste, dried, kept in *śarāva sampuṭa* and cooked in *gaja puṭa.* This process should be repeated for three times. Thereafter, it should be made to a fine powder by triturating in a pestle and mortar and kept in a dry air-tight glass bottle.

Therapeutic Indications

The *bhasma* of deer-horn is exceedingly useful in the treatment of heart diseases including angina pectoris, pleurisy and pain in the sides of the chest.

Dose

125 to 250 mg. twice daily in empty stomach.

Anupāna or Vehicle

Fresh butter, ghee, milk or honey.

ŚILĀ JATU (MINERAL PITCH)

Synonyms

Śaileya, śilāja, śaila dhātuja, śilāmaya, śilā sveda, śilā niryāsa, aśmaja, aśma jatuka, adrija, girija and *aśmottha.*

Śilā jatu (mineral pitch) is an exudate from stones in the mountains of high altitude. Because of the strong heat of the sun, some metallic contents of these stones get melted and come out. Normally, this exudate is eaten away by the animals and birds inhabiting the mountain. The exudate which comes out of the stone directly because of heat of the sun ray is, undoubtedly, the best for therapeutic purposes. Since it is rarely available, generally the stones from these mountains are collected, boiled in hot water and the scum over it is collected for medicinal use.

Adverse Effects of Impure Śilā Jatu

Impure *śilā jatu,* if used, may cause burning sensation all over the body, fainting, giddiness and *rakta pitta* (a disease characterised by bleeding from different parts of the body).

Purification

For purification of the *śilā jatu,* four iron trays are necessary. In one of these trays, the powder of *śilā jatu* or the stone producing *śilā jatu* should be kept. To this, double the quantity of hot water and half the quantity of *triphalā* (see Appendix I) decoction should be added. It should be kept in sun for three hours. Then it should be stirred well and the water filtered out. This water should be kept in one of these iron trays and exposed to hot sun. Because of the heat of the sun, scum will appear over the water. This has to be slowly taken out and collected in the second tray. To this, double the quantity of warm water should be added and stirred. When the water settles down, the scum will again appear over its surface which should be transferred to the third tray. Similarly, the scum of the third tray should be removed and collected in the fourth tray. This is the purified form of *śilā jatu.* This should be exposed to the sun, dried and stored in a glass bottle.

For purification of *śilā jatu,* it is necessary that the sun should be hot and there should be no wind. Care should be taken not to disturb the trays when the process of scum formation is taking place. The *śilā jatu* collected by this process is called *sūrya tāpī* (collected by the heat of sun). The other method, which is generally followed by big drug manufacturers, is to boil the stones of *śilā jatu* with the help of *triphalā* (see Appendix I) decoction and to filter the liquid. This liquid should be further boiled till it gets concentrated. Thereafter, this concentrated paste is exposed to sun rays for the *śilā jatu* to get dried up. This process is called *agni tāpī* (collected by the heat of the fire).

Testing

Since *śilā jatu* is a very popular and effective remedy, often it is adulterated in the market. Therefore, it should be tested to ascertain its purity before it is used. A small quantity of *śilā jatu* should be placed over a hot charcoal. If pure, no smoke will come out of it and the *śilā jatu* will take the shape of a cylinderical mass. It should be pungent and bitter in taste and it should have the smell of the cow's urine.

Another method of testing *śilā jatu* is to take a small quantity of it and place it over the surface of water. It will gradually sink to the bottom of the vessel in the form of stricks and it will not just get mixed up with the water.

Properties

Śilā jatu is bitter and pungent in taste, hot in potency, pungent in *vipāka,* diuretic, *yoga vāhin* (which enhances the property of another drug when added to the latter) and *rasāyana* or rejuvenating.

Therapeutic Indications

According to *Caraka saṃhitā,* there is no curable disease in this world which is not cured effectively by the use of *śilā jatu.* It promotes strength and it is useful in the treatment of oedema, anemia, tuberculosis, asthma, enlargement of spleen, chronic fever, epilepsy, schizophrenia, *prameha* (obstinate urinary disorders including diabetes), *udara* (obstinate abdominal diseases including ascites), stone in urinary tract, heart diseases, colic pain, vomiting, rheumatism, gout and diseases of nervous system. It is specifically useful in the treatment of stone in gall bladder. It has the property of increasing the compactness of the body. It is useful in reducing blood cholesterol and obesity. It helps in the healing of fracture and torn ligaments.

Precautions

No drug or diet, which reduces the compactness of the body, should be used along with *śilā jatu.* It is generally used in the treatment of stone in the urinary tract and gall bladder. Another drug, which is also used for this purpose, is *kulattha* (*Dolichos biflorus* Linn.). *Kulattha* is also used as a pulse for food. Modes of action of *śilā jatu* and *kulattha* are different inasmuch as *śilā jatu* breaks the stone into small pieces by which it comes out of the body and *kulattha* gradually dissolves the stone for its elimination. *Śilā jatu* makes the body compact and *kulattha* reduces the compactness. Therefore, these two drugs should not be used simultaneously.

Dose

250 mg. to 1 gm., two to three times per day.

Anupāna or Vehicle

Hot milk.

CHAPTER IX

POISONOUS VEGETABLE PRODUCTS

VATSANĀBHA (ACONITUM CHASMANTHUM STAFF EX HOLMES)

Synonyms

Vatsa nāga, kṣveḍa, viṣa and *amṛta.*

Botanically, several plants are used as *vatsa nābha.* Of these, *Aconitum chasmanthum* Staff ex Holmes is the most effective as medicine. It is the root of this plant which is used. Its root should be collected after the seeds of this plant are matured. Fresh root should be used in medicine. Old stock gets infested with insects and should not be used.

Part Used

Root.

Adverse Effects of Impure Aconite

If used without appropriate purification, it causes burning sensation all over the body, fainting, cardiac arrest and even death.

Purification

It should be washed with warm water to clean external impurities like mud and sand. It should be cut into small pieces of the size of peas and soaked in cow's urine for seven days. Every day, cow's urine should be replaced by fresh urine and during the day time, the container should be kept exposed to strong rays of the sun. After the seventh day, it should be again washed with warm water and its outer bark should be removed from these small pieces. Then these pieces are to be dried in the sun.

Testing

Before using aconite in medicine, the physician should ensure that the drug is absolutely free from toxicity. A small piece of this purified aconite should be placed over the tongue. If it is free from toxicity, then there will be no tingling sensation and numbness of the tongue. If these sensations are observed, then the aconite should be processed with cow's urine again.

Properties

It is pungent, astringent and bitter in taste, hot in potency, *yoga vāhin* (which enhances the properties of a drug when added to the latter), *rasāyana* (rejuvenating agent) and alleviator of all the three *doṣas.*

Therapeutic Indications

It is useful in the treatment of *agni māndya* (suppression of the power of digestion and metabolism), splenomegaly, rheumatism, gout, asthma, chronic bronchitis, piles, fistula-in-ano, sprue syndrome, *gulma* (phantom tumour), acute and chronic fever, *kuṣṭha* (obstinate skin diseases including leprosy), anemia, night blindness, conjunctivitis, otitis media, earache, headache, sciatica, lumbago and snake bite.

It is rarely used alone. Generally, it is given in combination with other drugs in a compound form. Externally, it is used in the form of medicated oils.

Dose

10 - 20 mg., twice daily.

Anupāna or Vehicle

Honey or milk.

Precautions

The patient using aconite should avoid heat producing food as well as drinks and alcohol. Borax and alum are antidotes of aconite poisoning.

VIṢA TINDUKA (STRYCHNOS NUX-VOMICA LINN.)

Synonyms

Kucelaka, kucela, kucilā, viṣa tindu, tindu, tinduka, kāraskara, ramya phala, kupāka, viṣa muṣṭikā and *kāla kūṭa.*

Part Used

Seeds.

Adverse Effects of Impure Nux-Vomica

Administration of nux-vomica without proper purification causes tetanic convulsions, muscular pain, excessive thirst and redness of skin.

Method of Purification

Seeds of nux-vomica should be tied in a piece of cloth and made to a *poṭṭalī*. It should be cooked in *Dolā yantra* for three hours by adding cow's milk. Seeds should then be washed with warm water. The outer coating of these seeds should be removed by scraping through a knife. Then, after drying in sun, these seed-kernels should be cut into small pieces and fried in cow's ghee. Then the powder should be prepared of these pieces and kept in a glass bottle for medicinal use.

Properties

Nux-vomica is pungent in taste and hot in potency. It stimulates digestion and virility. It reduces fat including cholesterol in the body. It is diuretic.

Therapeutic Indications

It is used in several aphrodisiac recipes. It is used in the treatment of sprue syndrome, schizophrenia, *agni māndya* (suppression of the power of digestion), gastritis, peptic ulcer, cardiac afflictions, asthma, pleurisy, facial paralysis, neuralgia, headache, lumbago and urinary disorders.

Dose

25 mg. to 125 mg. twice daily. It is generally used in combination with other drugs in a compound form.

Anupāna or Vehicle

Milk, ghee or butter.

Precautions

While taking nux-vomica, the patient should avoid heat producing diet and drinks. He should use more of cow's milk, butter and ghee. Cow's ghee is an antidote of nux-vomica poisoning.

JAYA PĀLA (CROTON TIGLIUM LINN.)

Synonyms

Jepāla, recaka, sāraka, vibhedanī and *mala drāvī.*

Parts Used

Seeds.

Adverse Effects of Impure Croton Seed

Croton seed is a strong purgative. If used without appropriate purification, it might cause excessive purging leading to dehydration, cramps, burning sensation and excessive thirst.

Method of Purification

Croton seed should be soaked in water for one night. Its outer coating should be removed. From inside the kernel, leaf like cotyledons should also be removed. Then these are to be tied in a piece of cloth in the form of a *poṭṭalī* (round bolus). It should then be cooked in *Dolā yantra* (see Appendix II) by adding cow's milk. Thereafter, these kernels should be removed from the *poṭṭalī,* washed with water and dried in the sun. To remove the residual oil, these kernels should be pressed through two blotting papers and stored in a dry and new earthen jar.

Properties

Croton seed is bitter in taste, pungent in *vipāka* (taste that emerges after digestion and during metabolism) and hot in potency. It is a strong purgative. It alleviates *vāyu* and *kapha.*

Therapeutic Indications

It is used in the treatment of ascites, cirrhosis of liver, intestinal parasites and *kuṣṭha* (obstinate skin diseases including leprosy).

Dose

15 mg. to 25 mg.

It is generally used in combination with other drugs in a compound form.

Anupāna or Vehicle

Cold water.

Precautions

If there is excessive purgation, to stop it, cold water should never be used. On the other hand, warm water will stop motions. Borax is an antidote of croton seed poisoning.

DHUSTŪRA (DATURA METEL LINN.)

Synonyms

Dhattūra, kitava, unmatta, dhūrta, svarṇa, kanaka, śaṭha, kaṇṭaka phala and *śiva śekhara.*

Parts Used

The entire plant of datura is used in medicine but its seeds are exceedingly potent as therapeutic agent, and these seeds should be used in medicine only after *śodhana* (purification).

Adverse Effects of Impure Datura

Datura, if used without appropriate *śodhana,* may cause dryness, excessive thirst, cramps, unconsciousness and giddiness.

Method of Purification

Seeds of datura should be cleaned of physical impurities and tied in a piece of cloth in the form of *poṭṭalī* (round bolus). It should be cooked in *Dolā yantra* (see Appendix II) by adding cow's urine or cow's milk for three hours. Thereafter, these seeds should be washed with warm water and dried in the sun.

Properties

Datura is pungent in taste, hot in potency and pungent in *vipāka* (the taste that emerges after digestion and during metabolism).

Therapeutic Indications

Datura is used in the treatment of oedema, asthma, bronchitis, fever, *kṛmi* (intestinal parasites) and *kuṣṭha* (obstinate skin diseases including leprosy), lumbago, earache, rheumatism, gout and colic pain.

Dose

25 mg. to 50 mg. It is generally used in combination with other drugs in a compound form.

Anupāna or Vehicle

Cow's milk.

BHAṄGĀ (CANNABIS SATIVA LINN.)

Synonyms

Bhaṅgā, bhaṅgī, mātulānī, mādinī, mātikā, mātulī, vijayā, tandrā kāriṇī and *bahu vādinī.*

Parts Used

Unpolinated inflorescence *(gāñjā)* and tender leaves including fruits *(bhāṅga)*.

Adverse Effects of Impure Bhaṅgā

If taken without appropriate *śodhana* (purification), it causes delirium, giddiness and unconsciousness.

Method of Purification

Bhaṅgā or *gāñjā* should be soaked in water for 24 hours. Then it should be squeezed out and dried. Thereafter, it should be fried in cow's ghee with mild fire and stored in a clean glass bottle.

Properties

Bhaṅgā is bitter in taste, hot in potency, constipative, digestive stimulant, carminative, alleviator of *kapha*, aggravator of *pitta* and intoxicating.

Therapeutic Indications

It is used in the treatment of impotency, sprue syndrome, chronic colitis, chronic dysenṭery, colic-pain, nephritis, headache, dysmenorrhea, depression, sleeplessness and piles.

Dose

250 mg. to 500 mg.

Anupāna or Vehicle

Milk added with sugar.

Precautions

In case of any adverse effect, the patient should be given lemon juice or tamarind to eat which counter-acts the intoxicating effect of *bhaṅgā*.

BHALLĀTAKA (SEMECARPUS ANACARDIUM LINN. F.)

Synonyms

Bhallāta, tapana, agni, vahni, dahana, vāyu sakhā, vātāri, vraṇakṛt, kṛmighna and *aruṣkara.*

Part Used

Seed.

Adverse Effects of Impure Bhallātaka

If used without proper *śodhana* (purification), *bhallātaka* causes blisters, glossitis, diarrhoea, menorrhagia, ulcers, oedema and burning sensation.

Method of Purification

The seed of *bhallātaka* should be soaked in water and rubbed over a piece of brick till the outer coating is removed. With the help of a knife, its top portion should be removed. Then it should be washed with warm water. Thereafter, these seeds should be tied in a piece of cloth in the form of *poṭṭalī* (round bolus) and cooked in *Dolā yantra* (see Appendix II) by adding cow's milk for three hours. Thereafter, these seeds should again be washed with warm water and dried.

Properties

Bhallātaka is pungent and bitter in taste, hot in potency, pungent in *vipāka* (taste that emerges after digestion and during metabolism) and *rasāyana* (rejuvenating).

Therapeutic Indications

It is useful in the treatment of *gulma* (phantom tumour), piles, splenic disorders, sprue syndrome, *kuṣṭha* (obstinate skin diseases including leprosy), *udara* (obstinate abdominal diseases including ascites), chronic constipation, colic-pain and asthma.

Dose

125 mg. to 500 mg.

Anupāna or Vehicle

Milk, butter or ghee.

Precautions

Some persons are very allergic to *bhallātaka*. They should not handle this drug during *śodhana* and such patients should never be given this drug.

Before using *bhallātaka* or its preparation, the mouth should be smeared with ghee, and if during the treatment by *bhallātaka* there is itching in the anus or urethra, salivation, gingivitis or glossitis, then the therapy should be discontinued. Coconut is a good antidote. Its pulp and water can be used to counter-act the toxic effects of *bhallātaka*.

GUÑJĀ (ABRUS PRECATORIUS LINN.)

Synonyms

Raktikā, raktā, tāmrikā, kṛṣṇa cūḍikā, uccaṭā, śīta pākī, bhilla bhūṣaṇikā, aruṇā, cūḍā maṇi, śikhaṇḍī, kṛṣṇalā, kākaṇantī and *kāmbhojī*.

Parts Used

Leaves, roots and seeds. Leaves and roots are non-toxic.

Adverse Effects of Impure Guñjā

If used without appropriate purification, *guñjā* causes vomiting and diarrhoea.

Method of Purification

Guñjā seeds should be crushed and tied in a piece of cloth in the form of a *poṭṭalī* (round bolus). It should be cooked in *Dolā yantra* (see Appendix II) by adding cow's milk for three hours. Then these seeds should be washed with warm water and dried.

Properties

Guñjā is bitter and pungent in taste and hot in pontency. It is aphrodisiac.

Therapeutic Indications

It is useful in the treatment of leucoderma, impotency and *ūrustambha* (stiffness of thighs). It is an oral contraceptive.

Dose

50 mg. to 150 mg., twice daily in empty stomach. If there is nausea or vomiting, then it can be used after food also.

Anupāna or Vehicle

Honey or milk.

APPENDIX I

PARIBHĀṢĀ OR GLOSSARY OF TECHNICAL TERMS

In *Rasa śāstra,* certain technical terms are often used. Explanation of these terms is called *paribhāṣā*. Those interested in the details of *Rasa śāstra* should be acquainted with the exact meaning of these technical terms some of which are already described in this work.

Lavaṇa Pañcaka (Five Salts)

Saindhava (rock-salt), *sāmudra* (sea-salt), *viḍa* (black salt containing Ammonium chloride), *sauvarcala* (sonchal salt containing iron and sulphur) and *romaka* (another type of salt)--these five taken together are called *pañca lavaṇa.*

Lavaṇa Traya (Three Salts)

Saindhava, sauvarcala and *viḍa* — these three salts taken together are called *lavaṇa traya.*

Kṣāra Dvaya (Two Alkalies)

Svarjī kṣāra (Sodium bicarbonate) and *yava kṣāra* (alkali preparation of barley ash containing Potassium bicarbonate and Potassium carbonate) — these two taken together are called *kṣāra dvaya.*

Kṣāra Traya (Three Alkalies)

Svarjī kṣāra, yava kṣāra and *saubhāgya* (borax)--these three taken together are called *kṣāra traya.*

Kṣāra Pañcaka (Five Alkalies)

Kṣāras (alkali preparations) of *kadalī* (*Musa paradisiaca* Linn.), *muṣkaka* (*pāṭalā=Stereospermum suaveolens* DC.), *kiṃśuka* (*Butea monosperma* Kuntze), *tila* (*Sesamum indicum* Linn.) and *svarjī kṣāra*— these five taken together are called *kṣāra pañcaka.*

Kṣārāṣṭaka (Eight Alkalies)

Kṣāras (alkali preparation) of *sudhā* (*Euphorbia neriifolia* Linn.), *palāśa* (*Butea monosperma* Kuntze), *apāmārga* (*Achyranthes aspera* Linn.), *ciñcā* (*Tamarindus indica* Linn.), *arka* (*Calotropis gigantea* R. Br. ex Ait.), *tila* (*Sesamum indicum* Linn.), *yava* (*Hordeum vulgare* Linn.) and *svarjī kṣāra* (*Sodium bicarbonate*) — these eight taken together are called *kṣārāṣṭaka.*

Mūtrāṣṭaka (Eight Types of Urine)

Urine of she buffalo, she goat, female sheep, cow, male camel, male ass, male elephant and horse--these eight taken together are called *mūtrāṣṭaka.*

Amla Varga (Group of Sour Drugs)

Jambīra (*Citrus limon* Burm. f.), *nimbūka* (*Citrus aurantifolia* Swingle), *amla vetasa* (*Garcinia pedunculata* Roxb.), *amlikā* (*Tamarindus indica* Linn.), *nāraṅga* (*Citrus reticulata* Blanc.), *dāḍima* (*Punica granatum* Linn.), *vṛkṣāmla* (*Garcinia indica* Chois.), *bīja pūraka* (*Citrus medica* Linn.), *cāṅgerī* (*Oxalis corniculata* Linn.), *caṇakāmla* (*Cicer arietinum* Linn.), *karkandhu* (*Zizyphus nummularia* W. & H.), *kara mardaka* (*Carissa carandas* Linn.) and *cukrīkā* (*Rumex vesicularis* Linn.)--these drugs taken together are called *amla varga.*

Amla Pañcaka (Five Sour Drugs)

Amla vetasa, jambīra, mātuluṅga (*bīja pūra*), *nāraṅga* and *nimbuka* — these five taken together are called *amla pañcaka.*

Kola (*Zizyphus jujuba* Lam.), *dāḍima* (*Punica granatum* Linn.), *vṛkṣāmla* (*Garcinia indica* Chois.), *cāṅgerī* (*Oxalis corniculata* Linn.) and *ciñcā* (*Tamarindus indica* Linn.) — these five drugs taken together are called *amla pañcaka.*

Pañca Tikta (Five Bitter Drugs)

Guḍūcī (*Tinospora cordifolia* Miers), *nimba* (*Azadirachta indica* A. Juss.), *vāsā* (*Adhatoda vasica* Nees), *kaṇṭakārī* (*Solanum xanthocarpum* Schrad. and Wendle.) and *paṭola* (*Trichosanthes cucumerina* Linn.) — these five drugs taken together are called *pañca tikta*.

Pañca Mṛttikā (Five Clays)

Powder of brick, ash, earth from ant-hill, *gairika* (red ochre) and salt--these five taken together are called *pañca mṛttikā*.

Madhura Traya (Three Sweet Drugs)

Ghee, jaggery and honey — these three taken together are called *madhura traya*.

Pañcāmṛta (Five Nectars)

Cow's milk, curd of cow's milk, cow's ghee, honey and sugar — these five taken together are called *pañcāmṛta*.

Pañca Gavya (Five Cow-Products)

Milk, curd, ghee, urine and dung of the cow — these five taken together are called *pañca gavya*.

Kṣīra Traya (Three Milky Latexes)

The latexes of *arka* (*Calotropis gigantea* R. Br. ex Ait.), *vaṭa* (*Ficus bengalensis* Linn.) and *snuhī* (*Euphorbia neriifolia* Linn.) — these three taken together are called *kṣīra traya*.

Dugdha Varga (Group of Milks)

Milk of she elephant, mare, cow, female sheep, she goat, she camel, she buffalo, she ass and woman and the milky latexes of *kākodumbara* (*Ficus hispida* Linn. f.), *snuhī* (*Euphorbia neriifolia* Linn.), *dugdhikā* (*Euphorbia hitra* Linn.), *udumbara* (*Ficus racemosa* Linn.), *arka* (*Calotropis gigantea* R. Br. ex Ait.), *nyagrodha* (*Ficus bengalensis*

Linn.), aśvattha (*Ficus religiosa* Linn.) and *tilvaka* (*Symplocos racemosa* Roxb.) — all these taken together are called *dugdha varga*.

Taila Varga (Group of Oils)

Oil of the seeds of *tila* (*Sesamum indicum* Linn.), *sarṣapa* (*Brassica comprestris* var. Sarson Prain.), *dhattūra* (*Datura metel* Linn.), *bhallātaka* (*Semecarpus anacardium* Linn. f.), *eraṇḍa* (*Ricinus communis* Linn.), *nimba* (*Azadirachta inidca* A. Juss.), *jaya pāla* (*Croton tiglium* Linn.), *dantī* (*Baliospermum montanum* Muell-Arg.), *kusumbha* (*Carthamus tinctorius* Linn.) and *umā* (*Linum usitatissimum* Linn.) — all these taken together are called *taila varga*.

Drāvaka Gaṇa (Melting Drugs)

Guñjā (*Abrus precatorius* Linn.), honey, jaggery, ghee, borax and *guggulu* (*Commiphora mukul* Engl.) — these taken together are called drāvaka *gaṇa*.

Divyauṣadhi Varga (Group of Celestial Drugs)

Soma vallī, soma vṛkṣa, sthala padminī, gonāśa, uccaṭa, īśvarī, bhuta keśi, kṛṣṇa lata, laśuna vallī, rudantī, vārāhī, sapta patrī, nāginī, sarpiṇī, chatriṇī, gośṛṅgī, jyotirlatā, rakta vallī, padma vallī, kākīṇī, cāṇḍālī, tāmra vallī, pīta vallī, vijayā, mahauṣadhi, deva dālī, navanītaka gandhī, garuḍa vallī, tumbinī, bhū tumbunī, gandharva, vyāghra pādī, mahauṣadhi (another variety), *gomārī, triśūlī, rutasī, tridaṇḍī, bhṛṅga vallī, camarikā, karavīra latā, vajra vallī, varā vallī, rohiṇī, bilvinī, gorocanā latā, karīrī, akṣara, apatrā, kuṭaja vallī, mūla kanda, brāhmaṇī, muni vallī, nimba vallī, tila kanda, atasī vallī, bodhi latā, madya gandhā, kūrma latā, mādhavī, viśālā, mahā nāga, mandaka latā, udumbara latā* and *citra vallī* — all these drugs taken together are called *divyauṣadhi varga*. Botanical identity of most of these drugs is shrouded in the mist of controversies. These drugs are known to saints living in the high Himalayas.

Biḍa (Catalytic Agent)

The recipe containing *kṣāras* (alkalies), *amlas* (sour drugs), *gandhaka* (sulphur), *mūtra* (urine) and salts, which is used for the assimilation of *bīja* (seed) by mercury, is called *biḍa*.

Mitra pañcaka (Five Friendly Drugs)

Ghee, *guñjā* (*Abrus precatorius* Linn.), borax, honey and *guggulu* (*Commiphora mukul* Engl.) — these five drugs taken together are called *mitra pañcaka*. They reduce the melting point of metals and minerals.

Gorvara (Cow-Dung Powder)

In the out-door cow-shed the dung gets dried up and because of the pressure of the hooves of cattle it becomes powder. This is called *gorvara*.

Kajjalī (Collyrium Like Powder)

If mercury, which is white and sulphur, which is yellow are triturated in a pestle and mortar without adding any liquid, it turns to a black powder. If sufficiently triturated, the powder becomes very fine like a collyrium preparation. This is called *kajjalī*.

Rasa Paṅka (Mud Like Preparation of Mercury)

If mercury and sulphur are triturated together by adding any liquid, then it becomes thin as well as soft and looks like black mud. This is called *rasa paṅka*.

Piṣṭikā (Paste)

If mercury and sulphur are triturated by adding milk, etc., then it becomes a thick paste like dough. It is called *rasa piṣṭī*.

Hiṅgulākṛṣṭa Rasa

Mercury collected from cinnabar by the process of sublimation is called *hiṅgulākṛṣṭa rasa*.

Dhātu Sattva (Essence of Metals)

If metals and minerals are triturated with drugs belonging to *drāvaka gaṇa*, kept inside a crucible and cooked in a *koṣṭhī* (fire place) attached with a blower, then the essence of the mineral comes out. This is called *dhātu sattva* or simply *sattva*.

Vanauṣadhi Sattva

The essence of herbs collected by distillation is called *vanaspati sattva* or *vanauṣadhi sattva.*

Siktha Taila

If bees wax and sesame oil, in equal quantities, are mixed together and heated in a pan, then the former melts and gets mixed up with the latter. When cooled, it becomes like butter. This is called *siktha taila.*

Āvāpa

Metals like tin, etc., melt when heated over fire in a pan. To this, the powder of drugs is added for reducing the metal to a *bhasma* form. This process is called *āvāpa* or *prativāpa.*

Nirvāpa, Niṣeka or Snāpana

Immersion of heated metal in liquids like water, etc., is called *nirvāpa, niṣeka* or *snāpana.*

Śuddhāvarta

When metal or mineral is kept in a crucible and heated strongly with the help of a blower in the fire place, the flame of the fire gradually becomes white and that is the stage which indicates the separation of *sattva* (essence). At this stage, the flame is called *śuddhāvarta.*

Ḍhālana

If the melted metal is poured into a liquid, the process is called *ḍhālana.*

Tāḍana

If the alloy of metals like bell-metal is strongly heated with the help of a blower to separate one metal from the other, it is called *tāḍana.*

Ghoṣākṛṣṭa

If the alloy of metals is mixed with drugs, which help in the separation of one of the ingredients (for example removal of tin from the bell-metal leaving copper alone) by heating strongly with the help of a blower, the process is called *ghoṣākṛṣṭa.*

Svataḥ Śīta

If the heated recipe is allowed to cool of its own over the oven or fire-place without removing the container from there, it is called *svāṅga śīta* or *svataḥ śīta.*

Bahiḥ Śīta

If the recipe is taken out of the oven or fire-place and then it cools down, it is called *bahiḥ śīta.*

Bhāvanā (Impregnation)

If a recipe is added with liquids and triturated till the latter dries up then the process is called *bhāvanā.* For this purpose, only that amount of the liquid should be added which will make the whole recipe wet and fill the container upto the upper level of the drug.

Śodhana (Purification)

Śodhana or purification of metals, minerals, gems, jewels or poisonous plants is done by adding drugs in various forms to them and then by triturating, cooking, ẹtc. This makes the substance non-toxic, easily digestible, assimilable and more effective therapeutically. This also makes the substance more fragile with a view to reduce it to a fine powder form by the process of *māraṇa.*

Māraṇa (Reduction to the State of Fine Powder)

Metals, minerals, gems and jewels are added with drugs in various forms and then cooked to reduce them to the state of fine powder. These are non-toxic and easily digestible as well as assimilable. They become therapeutically effective only in this condition. These powders are also called *bhasma.*

Piṣṭī (Making Powder Without Application of Heat)

Some gems and jewels are reduced to powder form by adding

liquids and triturating in a pestle and mortar. This is called *piṣṭī*. They have more cooling effect than *bhasmas*.

Amṛtīkaraṇa (Conversion into Nectar)

Some poisonous metals do not give up their toxic effects completely even after *śodhana* and *māraṇa*. They are further processed by adding more drugs till they become absolutely free from any toxic effect. This process is called *amṛtī karaṇa* or inculcation of the properties of nectar to the drug.

Vāritara (Floating over Water)

When the *bhasma* of a metal or mineral is properly prepared, it is tested to ascertain its quality. One of such tests is done by spreading the powder over the surface of water in a container. If the metal particles do not sink because of the gravitational force i.e. weight, but floats over the surface of water because of surface tension, then it is considered to be of good quality. This test is called *vāritara* or floating over water.

Rekhā Pūraṇa (Filling up Crevices of Finger)

The second method for testing a *bhasma* is to rub a small part of it between two fingers, and if the *bhasma* is properly prepared, then the powder should get filled in the crevices of the finger and no residue left. This is called *rekhā pūraṇa*.

Apunarbhava or Niruttha (Non-revival to the Original State)

If a *bhasma* is properly prepared then by adding drugs called *mitra pañcaka* (five drugs which reduce the melting point of metals) and cooking in a strong heat, it does not get converted into the original state of the metal. This is one of the tests employed to ascertain the quality of a *bhasma* and it is called *apunarbhava* or *niruttha*.

Dhanvantari Bhāga (Share of the Physician)

If a physician is employed to supervise the preparation of a recipe in the house of a private individual, then in exchange of his free labour he is entitled to a share of the medicine. This varies according to the nature of the recipe as follows :

	Nature of Preparation	Supervising Physician's Share
1.	Mercurial preparations, medicated ghees and medicated oils	½
2.	*Bhasma* of metals, minerals, gems and jewels	1/4th
3.	Linctus & syrup	1/8th
4.	Alcoholic preparations	1/4th
5.	Powders of vegetable drugs	1/7th

This share of the physician is called *Dhanvantari bhāga.* If the physician aspires or actually takes more than his share, it is considered unethical or a professional misconduct.

Parpaṭī (Scale Preparation)

The collyrium like powder of purified mercury and purified sulphur is used alone or in combination with other drugs in several categories of recipes. After melting, ingredients are kept over a piece of banana-leaf spread over the paste of cow-dung. With another leaf and cow-dung paste, pressure is applied from outside. The scale preparation, thus made out, is called *parpaṭī.*

Triphalā (Three Fruits)

Collective name of fruits of *harītakī* (*Terminalia chebula* Retz.), *bibhītakī* (*Terminalia belerica* Roxb.) and *āmalakī* (*Emblica officinalis* Gaertn.). Generally, the pulp of these fruits is used in medicine and taken in equal quantities. One fruit of *harītakī,* two fruits of *bibhītakī* and four fruits of *āmalakī* constitute one unit of *triphalā.*

Trikaṭu (Three Pungent Drugs)

Collective name for *śuṇṭhī* (*Zingiber officinale* Roscoe), *pippalī* (*Piper longum* Linn.) and *marica* (*Piper nigrum* Linn.), taken in equal quantities, is called *trikaṭu.*

APPENDIX II

EQUIPMENTS AND IMPLEMENTS USED IN RASA ŚĀSTRA

Some crucibles, ovens (fire place), *puṭas* and *yantras* (equipments) are specifically needed for the processing of metals and minerals. An outline of these items is given below :

A. MŪṢĀ (CRUCIBLE)

Mūṣās or crucibles are used for keeping metals, minerals, gems and jewels and heating them over strong fire. These containers are thermostable. Depending upon their requirements, these are prepared in different shapes with different ingredients as follows :

Sāmānya Mūṣā (Crucibles for General Use)

Charcoal, ash of the paddy husk, fibres of *śaṇa* (*Crotalaria juncea* Linn.) and horse-dung are taken together and mixed well by pounding with a hammer. A cone or funnel shaped crucible prepared of this material is called *sāmānya mūṣā* (crucible for general use). If any specific type of crucible is not prescribed, then this general type of crucible is used in the pharmaceutical process. If it is used for mixing two metals by melting together, then it is called *dvandva melāpana mūṣā*.

SĀMĀNYA MŪṢĀ (ORDINARY CRUCIBLE)

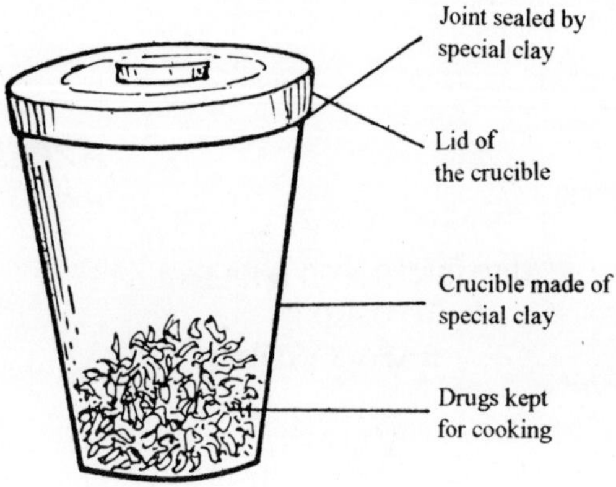

FIGURE - 1

Vajra Mūṣā

Three parts of clay (generally mud which is sandy, yellowish white in colour and composed of big particles is used), one part of *śaṇa,* one part of horse-dung, one part of ash of paddy husk and half part of *maṇḍūra* (iron rust)—all these are taken together and pounded well. The crucible prepared out of this is called *vajra mūṣā.* It is very strong and is used for taking out *sattva* (essence) of extremely hard substances like diamond.

Yoga Mūṣā

Ash of paddy husk, earth of white ant-hill, alkalies, sour liquids and salts are used in the preparation of clay for this type of crucible. This *yoga mūṣā* is used for preparing the *bhasma* of mercury.

Vajra Drāvaṇikā Mūṣā

Dried earth-worm, straw, ash of paddy-husk, etc., are taken in equal quantities and triturated with buffalo-milk. The crucible, prepared out of this clay, is called *vajra drāvaṇikā mūṣā.* It can easily stand six hours of strong heat.

Gāra Mūṣā

Black-soil (one part) and ash of paddy-husk (six parts) should be mixed with adequate quantities of *maṇḍūra* (iron rust), *śaṇa*, etc., and used for the preparation of the crucible. This is called *gāra mūṣā*.

Gostanī Mūṣā

The crucible prepared according to the size and in the shape of the nipple of cow is called *gostanī mūṣā*. It is generally used for taking out *sattva* (essence) of mica, etc. It is used with a lid. If it is shaped like the flower of *dhattūra* (*Datura metel* Linn.), it is called *dhustūra puṣpa mūṣā*.

GOSTANĪ AND DHUSTŪRA PUṢPA MŪṢĀ
(COW-NIPPLE LIKE AND DATURA FLOWER LIKE CRUCIBLES)

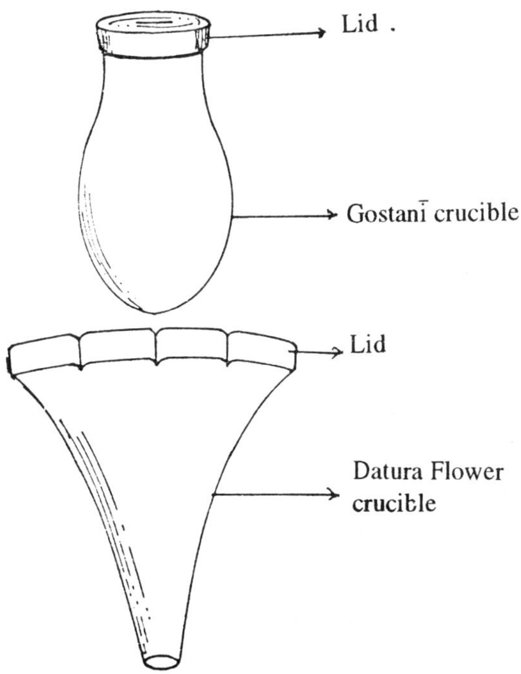

FIGURE - 2

Malla Mūṣā

If two round crucibles are kept face to face and used for the preparation of recipes, it is called *malla mūṣā.*

MALLA MŪṢĀ
(APPARATUS PREPARED OF TWO CRUCIBLES)

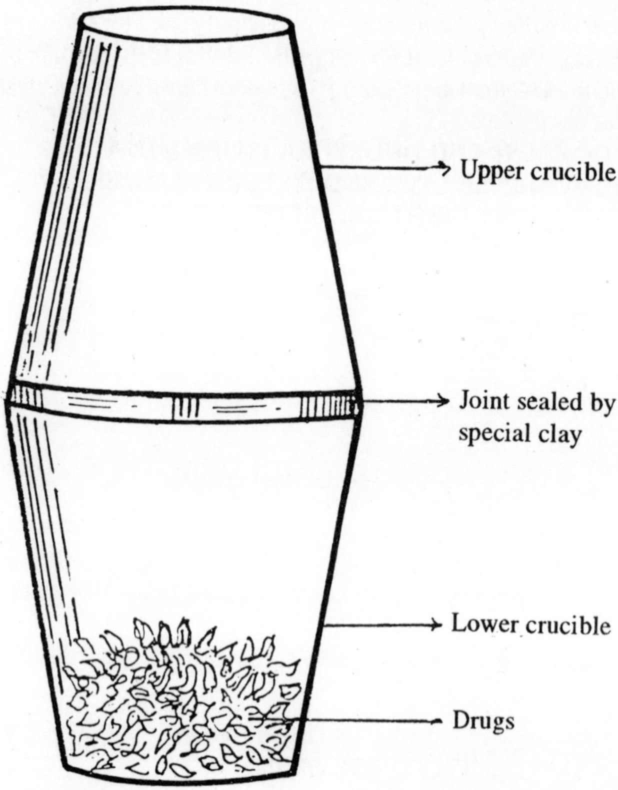

FIGURE - 3

Mahā Mūṣā

The crucible, which is big in size, having a wide mouth and a flat as well as round bottom, is called *mahā mūṣā.*

Vṛntāka Mūṣā

A crucible of 6" length and 2" breadth and having the shape of a brinjal (fruit of egg plant) should be prepared. It should have a hole at the top and through this, a lid of the shape of *dhattūra* flower having wide mouth and 4" tube should be inserted. This is called *vṛntāka mūṣā.*

VṚNTĀKA MŪṢĀ
(BRINJAL SHAPED CRUCIBLE)

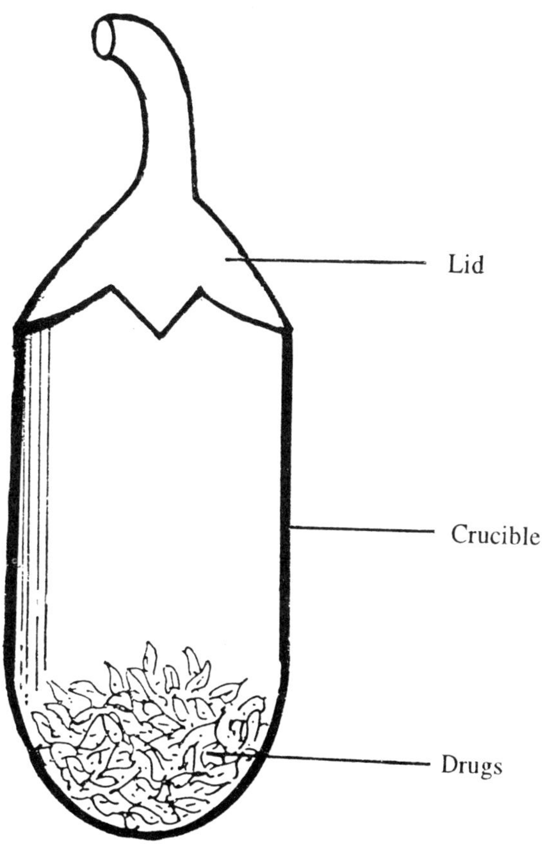

FIGURE - 4

B. KOṢṬHĪ (OVEN OR SPECIALLY PREPARED FIRE-PLACE)

In *Rasa śāstra* several types of fire-places or ovens are used for processing metals, etc. *Koṣṭhī* is a specialised fire-place where strong heat could be applied with the help of a leather blower. These are of several types. Two of them which are frequently used are described below :

Aṅgāra Koṣṭhikā

This is constructed above the ground. With the help of bricks, a wall should surround this fire place. It is 3' high and 1½' in length as well as breadth. The inside wall of this oven should be smeared with mud so that the heat of the fire inside does not come out. At the bottom of this oven a round hole of 2" diameter should be prepared to which the metal pipe connected with the leather blower should be inserted and the space around the tube in the hole should be sealed with mud. Charcoal or ordinary coal is ignited inside, and the crucible should be placed in an appropriate manner. With the help of the blower more heat should be produced. This is called *aṅgāra koṣṭhikā.*

AṄGĀRA KOṢṬHIKĀ
(SPECIAL TYPE OF OVEN)

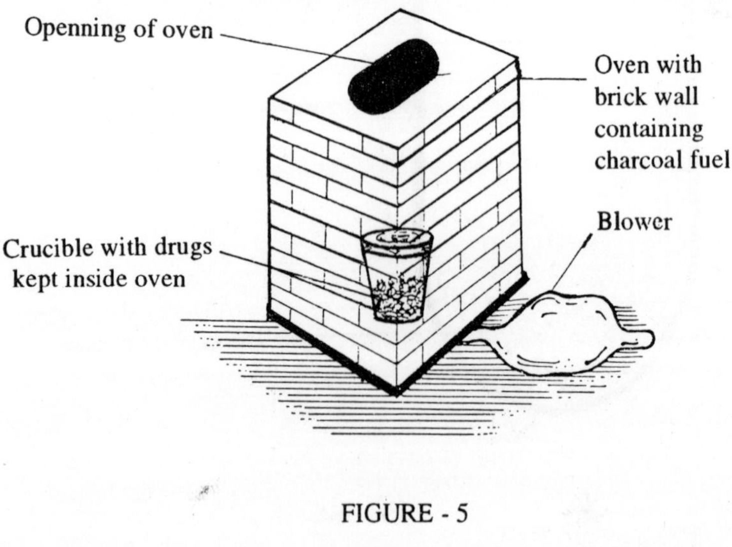

FIGURE - 5

Pātāla Koṣṭhikā

It is constructed underground. A pit of 6" height, 6" length and 6" breadth should be dug out. At the centre in the bottom another hole should be dug out. A pipe should be inserted into this hole from the outside ground near the pit and this pipe should be connected to a leather blower. The crucible is kept inside the pit and surrounded with coal. This is ignited. When blown from outside, it produces strong heat which enables the metal kept inside the crucible to melt. This is called *pātāla koṣṭhikā.*

PĀTĀLA KOṢṬHIKĀ
(UNDER-GROUND OVEN)

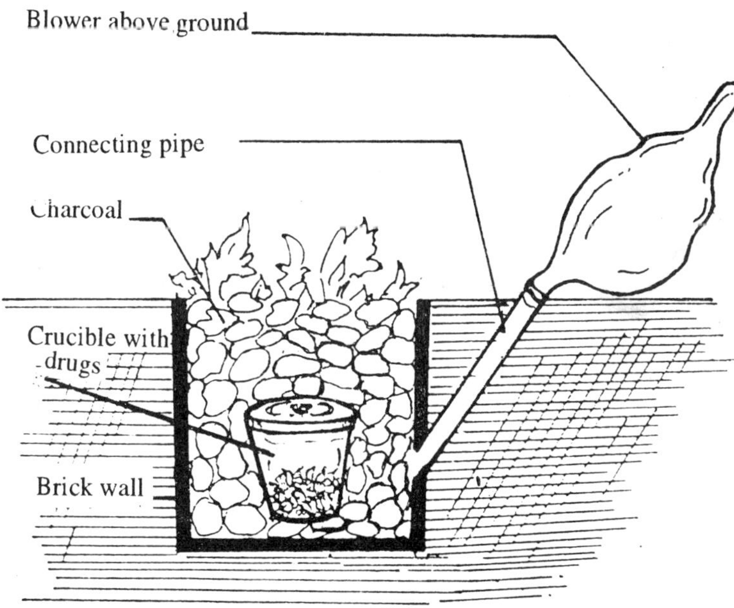

FIGURE - 6

C. PUṬA (OVEN OR FIRE-PLACE)

Different types of metals, minerals, gems and jewels need application of different amount of heat to be reduced to *bhasma* form. They are cooked in a specially designed fire-place which is called *puṭa*. Depending upon the heat requirement, some of them are arranged in pits of different sizes dug in the earth and some others are done over the ground. Cow-dung cake is generally used as fuel. Metals, etc., are kept inside two earthen plates (*śarāva sampuṭa*) put face to face and the joint sealed with the help of seven layers of mud-smeared cloth. Before cooking, this sealed container is well dried. The main purpose of the *puṭa* is to cook the material with the required quantity of heat constantly for a sufficient period. Once ignited, all the cow-dung cakes should be allowed to burn. When the fire is over, and the fire place is cooled down, the container should be removed. The layers of mud smeared cloth which were used for sealing the joint should then be scrapped and two plates separated to remove the metal, etc., inside for further processing. Some important types of *puṭa* are described hereafter.

Mahā Puṭa

The pit should be 42" deep, 36" long and 36" broad. This should be filled up with cow-dung cakes till half of its capacity. The container should be kept below the surface of it and the remaining portion of the pit should be filled up with more of cow-dung cakes. Thereafter, it should be ignited. This is called *mahā puṭa*.

MAHĀ PUṬA
(UNDER GROUND HEARTH FOR COOKING METALS)

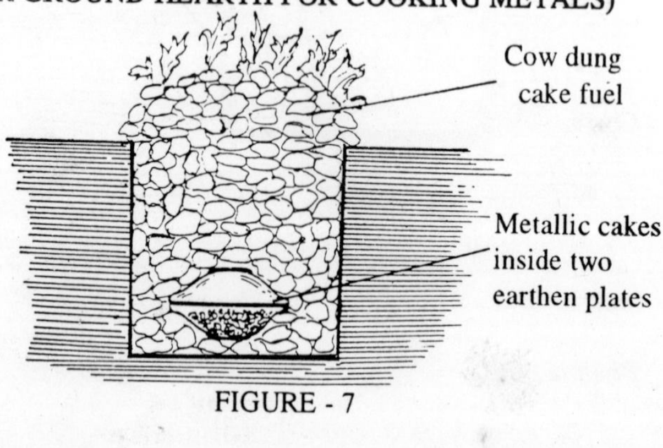

FIGURE - 7

Gaja Puṭa

The pit should be 22" in depth, length and breadth. It should be filled up with cow-dung cakes till half of its capacity and the container should be kept there. Then the remaining portion of the pit should be filled up with more cow-dung cakes and ignited. This is called *gaja puṭa*. If the pit is half of the above mentioned size, then it is called half *gaja puṭa* or *ardha gaja puṭa.*

Vārāha Puṭa

The pit should be 10" in depth, length and breadth. It should be filled up with cow-dung cakes till half and the container should be kept at that level. Then the remaining portion of the pit should be filled up with the cow-dung cakes and ignited. This is called *vārāha puṭa.*

Kukkuṭa Puṭa

The pit should be 6" in depth, length and breadth. It should be filled up with cow-dung cakes and the *śarāva sampuṭa* or container should be kept in the centre of the pit (in the middle). Then it should be ignited. This is called *kukkuṭa puṭa.*

Some physicians prefer to keep the container over the ground, cover it with the required amount of cow-dung cakes and ignite it.

Kapota Puṭa

A small pit should be dug out in the earth and the container should be kept in it. Over it, eight cow-dung cakes should be kept and ignited. This is called *kapota puṭa.*

Gorvara Puṭa

If a small earthen jar is filled up with cow-dung cakes, the container is kept in the middle of it and then ignited, it is called *gorvara puṭa.* It can also be done over the ground by putting a few cow-dung cakes, keeping the container in the middle and then igniting it.

Bhāṇḍa Puṭa

An earthen pot should be filled up with paddy-husk till half of its capacity. Over that, the container of the recipe should be kept and then the remaining portion of the pot should be filled up with paddy-husk. This should then be ignited. This is called *bhāṇḍa puṭa.*

BHĀṆḌA PUṬA
(COOKING INSIDE A JAR)

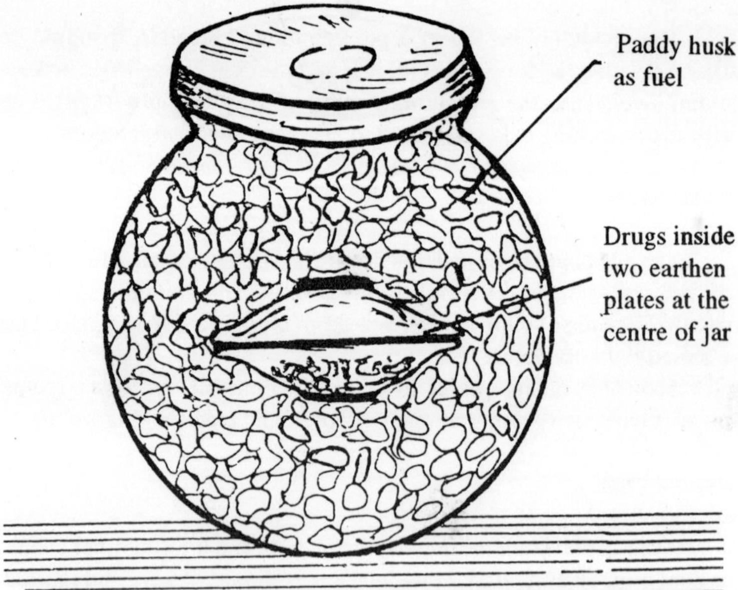

FIGURE - 8

Vāluka Puṭa

The crucible containing the material should be kept inside hot sand. This method is called *vālukā puṭa.*

Bhūdhara Puṭa

In a small pit dug under ground, the crucible containing the recipe should be kept, and on all sides, it should be surrounded by one inch of sand. Over the surface, fire should be applied. This type of cooking is called *bhūdhara puṭa.*

D. YANTRA (EQUIPMENT)

For the purification and *māraṇa* of metals, minerals, gems and jewels, various types of equipments are used. Some of these specially designed equipments are also used for the preparation of medicines out of metals, etc. These equipments can be prepared by clay, iron or stainless steel. Some of these commonly used equipments are described hereafter.

Dolā Yantra

The metal which is required to be cooked is wrapped with a piece of cloth. If mercury is to be cooked, then the cloth should be thick or it should be folded four times of wrapping. The mercury should be kept over a piece of *bhūrja patra* (*Betula utilis* D. Don.) or banana-leaf surrounded by the paste of drugs prescribed for the purpose and then tied by wrapping the cloth *(poṭṭalī).* This cloth should be hanged through a string from a stick or rod kept over a jar in such a way that no part of the cloth should touch either the sides or the bottom of the container. Then the jar should be filled up with the liquid prescribed for the purpose till it reaches upto half of the level of the *poṭṭalī*. Thus, the lower half of the *poṭṭalī* remains immersed in the liquid.

The container should then be placed over the fire. As the boiling starts, the level of liquid will go down. Periodically, therefore, more of the liquid should be added to the container or the *poṭṭalī* should be brought downwards so that it always remains immersed in the liquid upto half of its level. Some physicians prefer to cover the jar with a lid so that the evaporated moisture falls down after being condensed and there is very little loss of the fluid. In this way, boiling should continue till the prescribed period. Thereafter, the jar should be taken out of the fire, cooled and the *poṭṭalī* should be removed from the liquid. It should then be untied, the metal should be washed with warm water and dried up by keeping in the sun. This is called *Dolā yantra.*

DOLĀ YANTRA
(APPARATUS FOR COOKING IN LIQUID)

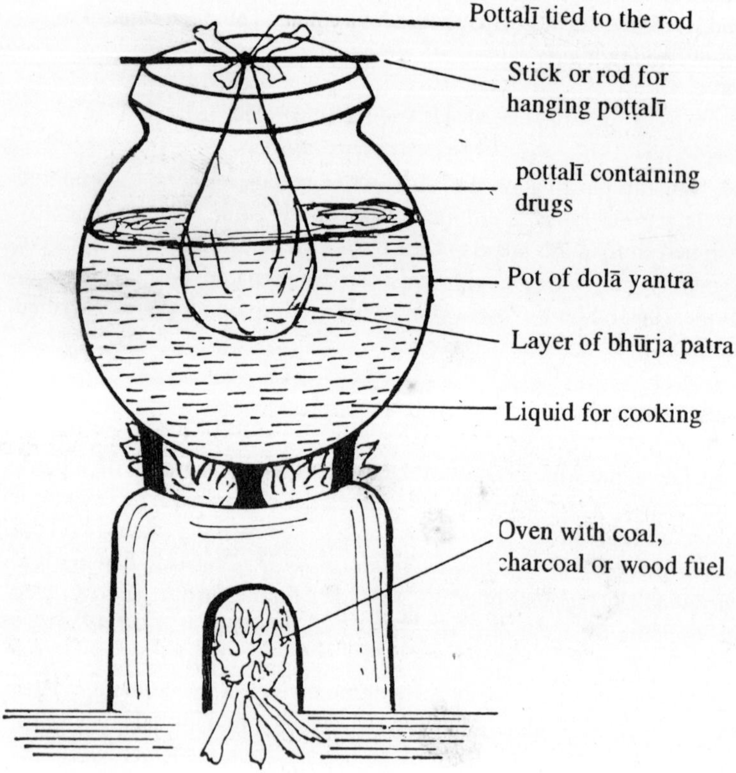

FIGURE - 9

Ūrdhva Pātana or Vidyādhara Yantra

This equipment is generally used for sublimation of mercury. It needs two earthen jars. In the lower jar, the paste of mercury triturated with prescribed drugs is kept. The mouth of this lower jar should be at least 6" in diameter. Over this, the second jar should be kept with its bottom down so that it protrudes inside the mouth of the lower jar. The point between these two jars should be carefully sealed with seven layers of mud smeared cloth and dried. Then it is kept over fire and the upper jar is filled with cold water. As a result of the heat of the fire, the water of the upper jar will become gradually warm. It should be continuously replaced by cold water to ensure that the bottom of the upper jar always remains cold. Because of the heat, mercury placed at the bottom of the lower jar will evaporate but it will get condensed at the bottom of the upper jar because of low temperature. After the prescribed period, fire should be extinguished and when completely cooled, the seal between the two jars should be broken carefully by scraping. Then, from the bottom of the upper jar, the sublimed mercury should be carefully removed by scraping through a knife. It should then be washed and dried. This is called *Ūrdhva pātana yantra* or *Vidyādhara yantra.*

ŪRDHVA PĀTANA YANTRA
(APPARATUS FOR SUBLIMATION)

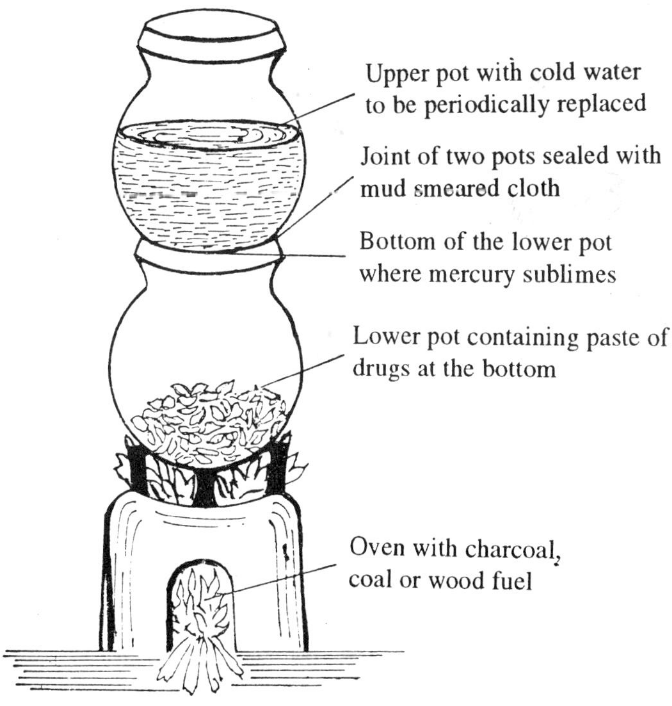

FIGURE - 10

Adhaḥ Pātana Yantra

For this equipment, two jars are required--one should be bigger than the other. The neck of the smaller jar should be narrow enough to protrude into the mouth of the bigger jar and remain fixed. Dig a pit in the earth which should be of the size of the bigger jar and the jar should be kept in it and filled with cold water up to the neck or at least upto half of its capacity. The inner surface of the smaller jar should be smeared with the mixture of mercury and the paste of drugs and dried. Then, it should be placed over the lower jar in an inverted position so that the neck of the former goes into the mouth of the lower jar and the joint between the two jars should be sealed with seven layers of mud smeared cloth to prevent evaporation of mercury while heating. It should be ensured that this sealed joint is just at the level of the ground or slightly below it. Then the upper jar should be covered with fuel and ignited. The fire should continue till the prescribed period. Generally, cow-dung cake is used for fuel. The mercury smeared in the inner wall of the upper jar will, thus, vaporise and come down. When it comes into contact with the cold water, kept in the lower jar, it condenses and gets accumulated at the bottom. When cooled, the seal at the joint between two jars should be broken by scraping and the upper jar gradually lifted. The lower jar should be taken out of the pit and the water decanted. The mercury deposited at the bottom should be washed and dried.

This equipment, which is generally used for the downward sublimation of mercury, is called *Adhaḥ pātana yantra.*

ADHAḤ PĀTANA YANTRA
(APPARATUS FOR DOWNWARD SUBLIMATION)

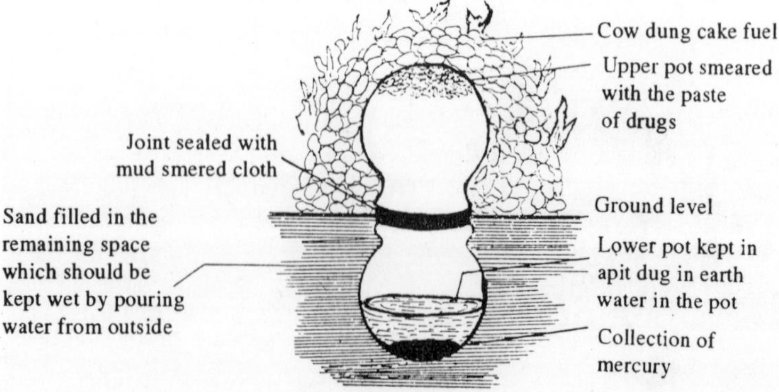

FIGURE - 11

Tiryak Pātana Yantra

This equipment is generally used for the distillation of mercury to make it free from impurities. For this, two jars with long necks are required. One of them is kept over the fire-place. The mercury along with the paste of drug is kept at the bottom of this jar. Near the neck of this jar, a hole is made to which a bamboo or glass or metallic tube is inserted. The second jar is kept at a lower level inside a pan full of water. The joint between the bamboo tube and the jar is carefully sealed not to allow any vapour to go out during the process of distillation. The jar containing mercury is heated and the vaporised mercury is collected through the bamboo or metallic or glass tube in the second jar kept inside a pan filled with cold water. It should be ensured that the water inside the pan does not become hot. If so, it should be replaced by cold water as and when required. Some cold water should be continuously poured over the surface of the second jar. It should be ensured that the mouths of both the jars are properly sealed to prevent any vapour coming out from the joints. The mercury after vaporisation will collect in the second jar and when it stops coming, the lower jar should be removed and the mercury should be collected from inside. It should then be washed and dried.

TIRYAK PĀTANA YANTRA
(APPARATUS FOR DISTILLATION)

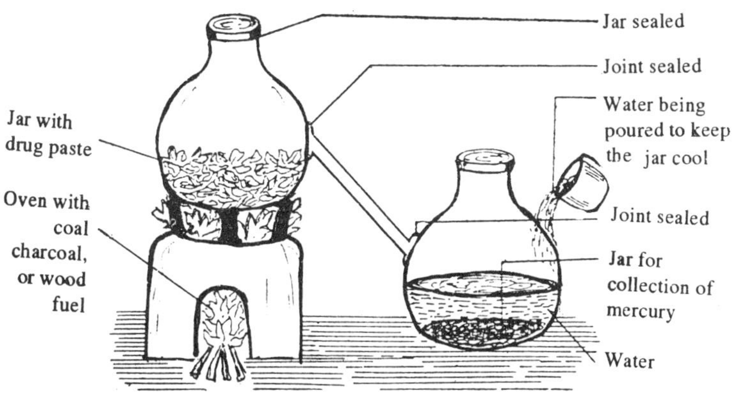

FIGURE - 12

This is called *Tiryak pātana yantra.* Now a days, several modern distilling apparatus are used in the place of the traditional equipments described before.

TIRYAK PĀTANA YANTRA (MODERN)
(MODIFIED APPARATUS FOR DISTILLATION)

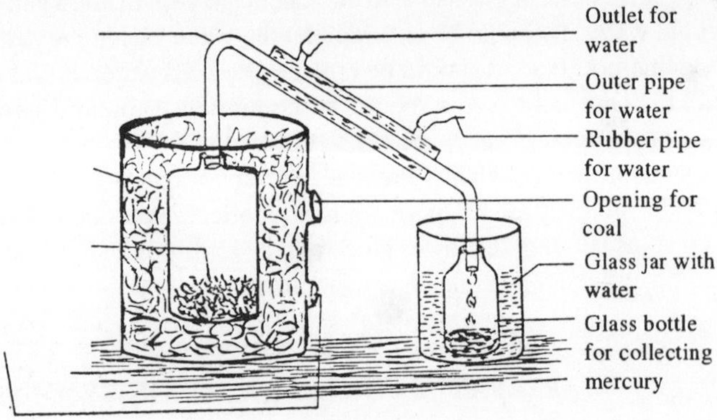

FIGURE - 13

Bhasma Yantra

This is generally used for making *bhasma* of arsenic, etc., which vaporises at a low heat. An earthen pot of 6" diameter, having a wide mouth, is used for this purpose. Half of this pot is filled with the ash and arsenic-cakes are placed over it. It is covered with another earthen plate having the same size at the mouth of the pot and the joint is sealed. Then, the pot is placed over fire and cooked for the prescribed period. When cooled, the seal should be opened and cakes of arsenic are carefully removed for further processing. This is called *Bhasma yantra.*

Kacchapa Yantra

This equipment is used for the *jāraṇā* (a special type of cooking) of mercury with sulphur. For this, two earthen or iron jars are required—one big and the other small. But their brims should be of the same size and shape. The big jar should be kept stable over the ground by providing adequate support at the bottom. It should be filled with water till 3/4th of its capacity. Over that, the other jar should be placed so that its bottom is within the water and the brim is over the brim of the lower pan. Sulphur and mercury, in the form of collyrium like powder, are kept in the upper pan. It should be ensured that the portion of the upper jar containing the powder of mercury and sulphur is already inside the water contained in the lower jar. Over the powder of the mercury and sulphur another earthen plate is kept with its face downwards to completely cover the whole of the powder and the joint is well sealed. Over this earthen plate, charcoal prepared out of wood of *khadira* (*Acacia catechu* Willd), should be kept and ignited till the entire sulphur is burnt. This is called *Kacchapa yantra*. This is generally used by physicians for the process of *jāraṇā* (literally digestion) of sulphur.

KACCHAPA YANTRA
(TORTOISE OR FLOATING APPARATUS)

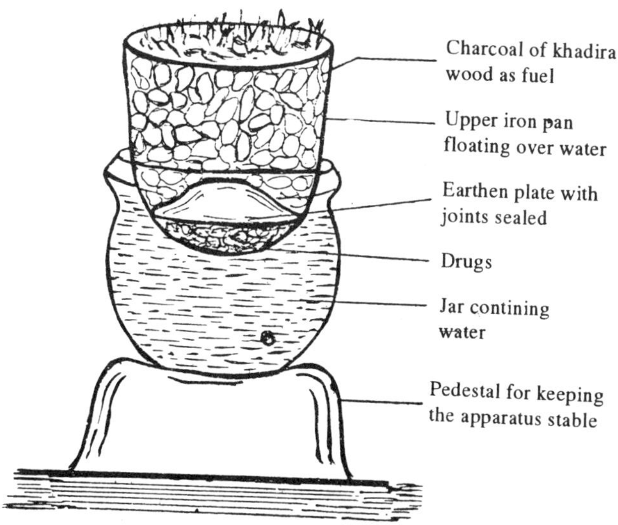

FIGURE - 14

Bhūdhara Yantra

In an earthen vessel having open mouth, one inch of sand should be kept. Over this sand, the crucible containing mercury should be kept. All around this crucible one inch of sand should be spread. Over it, cow-dung cakes should be kept. These cow-dung cakes should be ignited. This is called *Bhūdhara yantra*. Alternatively, a pit should be dug in the earth and covered with one inch of sand over which the crucible should be kept. This should be surrounded by one inch of sand. Over this, cow-dung cakes should be kept and ignited.

BHŪDHARA YANTRA
(APPARATUS FOR UNDER GROUND COOKING)

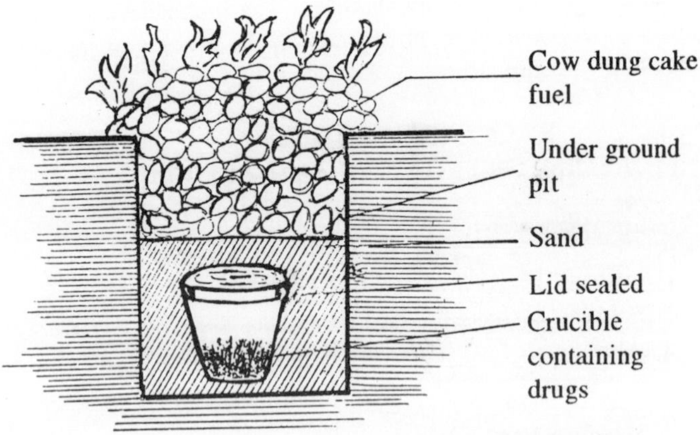

FIGURE - 15

Vāluka Yantra and Lavaṇa Yantra

The powdered mercury and sulphur should be kept inside a glass bottle which is strong and thermostable. This should be wrapped (except its mouth) with seven layers of mud-smeared cloth and dried. This bottle should be kept inside an earthen vessel, 10" in depth and having the mouth 10" in diameter. There should be a small hole (about 1/2" diameter) at the bottom of this jar which should be covered with a copper plate over which the bottle should be kept. The bottle then should be filled up upto 1/3rd of its capacity by the powder of purified mercury and purified sulphur *(kajjalī)*. The space between the bottle and wall of the earthen jar should be filled up with sand or salt. According to the prescribed procedure, heat should be applied from below by keeping the earthen vessel over a specially designed oven.

VĀLUKĀ YANTRA OR LAVAṆA YANTRA

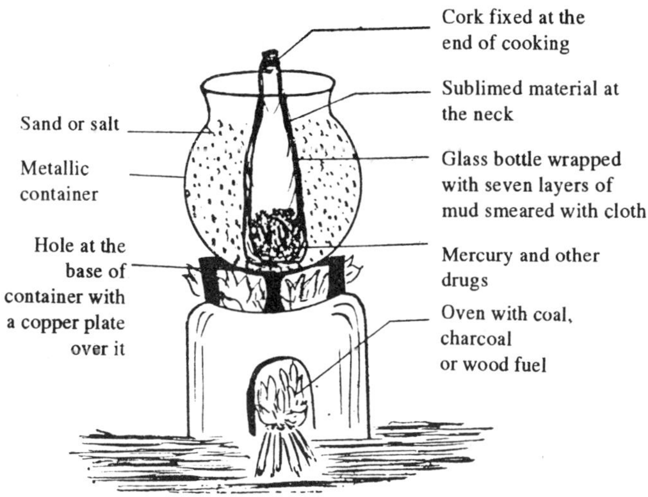

FIGURE - 16

In the beginning, the heat should be very mild. The fume of sulphur and even sulphur particles will gradually start coming out from the neck or the open mouth of the bottle. Then moderate heat should be applied and the neck of the bottle should be kept clean by periodically inserting a hot iron rod into it. If the mouth of the bottle gets blocked, then because of the pressure of the fume or vapour of sulphur, the whole glass bottle may explode. From the fume that comes out of the mouth of the bottle, the physician should ascertain the time when all the excess sulphur (which did not combine with mercury) gets evaporated. Thereafter, there is a possibility of the mercury vapour coming out. If a copper coin is placed near the mouth of the bottle then the mercury vapour, if coming out, will stick to the copper coin and give it a white colour. This stage should be avoided and before this stage is reached, the neck of the bottle should be covered with a cork and sealed with the help of seven layers of mud smeared cloth. Thereafter, the heat should be further intensified.

For each preparation, the amount of heat that should be applied in the beginning, in the middle and at the end is described. After the cooking is over, the earthen jar should be left over the oven to cool down. Thereafter, the bottle should be taken out and broken to collect the sublimed mercury-sulphur compound at its neck.

It is possible that a portion of the mercury-sulphur mixture along with other ingredients is left at the bottom of the bottle. This has to be cooked again. This is called *Vālukā yantra.*

If, in the place of sand, salt is kept inside the earthen vessel, then this is called *Lavaṇa yantra.*

Svedana Yantra

Two earthen vessels of equal size should be acquired for this purpose. In one of them, water or decoction or juice of herbs as specified in the recipe should be kept till half of its capacity. The brim of this vessel should be covered with a cloth or iron gauze and tied to the brim very firmly. Over this cloth, medicines required to be fomented should be kept. Over it, a second earthen vessel should be kept with its face downwards and the brims of both the vessels which are face to face should be sealed by mud smeared cloth. Heat should be applied by keeping both the vessels over an oven. This makes the liquid inside the lower vessel to evaporate, penetrate through the cloth and circulate in the upper vessel. Thus, the medicine kept over the cloth gets fomented. This is called *Svedana yantra*

SVEDANA YANTRA
(APPARATUS FOR STEAM-FOMENTATION)

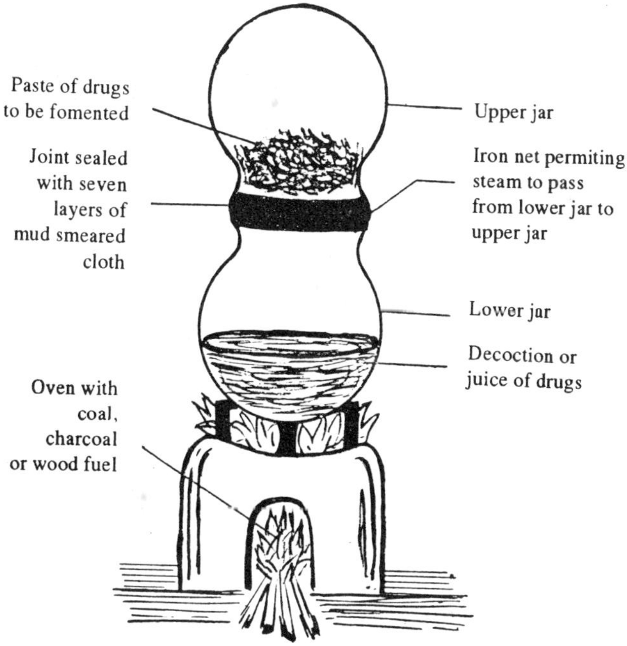

FIGURE - 17

Nāḍikā Yantra

The earthen jar with its mouth closed and with an opening in the side of its neck should be selected for this purpose. To this side opening, a tube should be fixed. This tube should then pass through water contained in a tray and its next opening should be into another bottle.

This equipment is generally used for distillation. Drugs are kept inside the jar along with some water. The jar is kept over an oven and heat is applied. Because of the heat, volatile fraction of the drug gets evaporated and passes through the tube. When it comes into contact with water, it cools down and gets collected in the bottle in the form of liquid. This is called *Nāḍikā yantra.*

NĀḌIKĀ YANTRA
(APPARATUS FOR EXTRACTION OF ARKA)

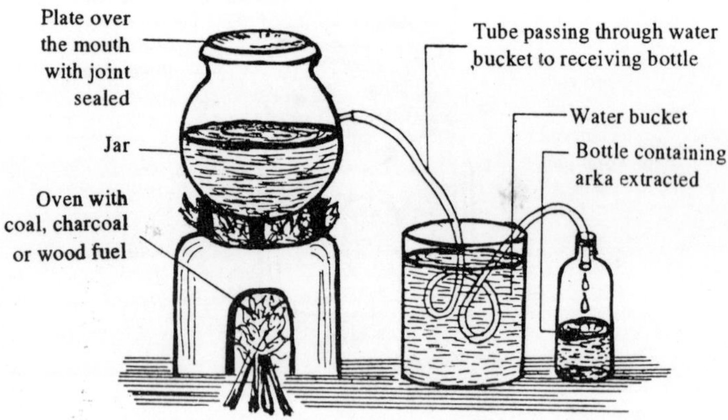

FIGURE - 18

Ḍamaru Yantra

Two earthen vessels of the same size are collected for this purpose. In one of them, drugs like mercury, sulphur and arsenic are kept. The other earthen vessel is placed over the first one with its face downwards. Brims of both these vessels are sealed by mud-smeared cloth. It is kept over an oven for cooking. Because of its dumb-bell like shape, it is called *Damaru yantra.*

ḌAMARU YANTRA
(DUMB-BELL LIKE APPARATUS)

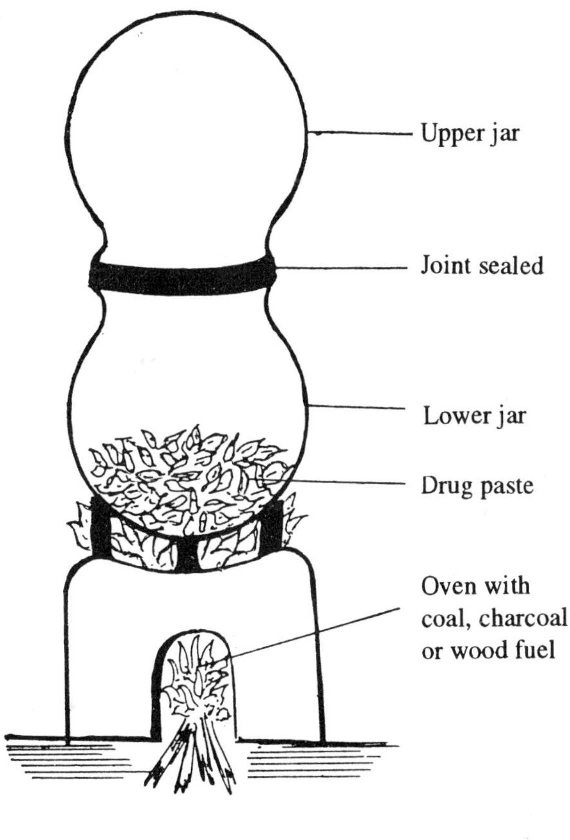

FIGURE - 19

Pātāla Yantra

A pit of about 2' in depth should be dug out. At the bottom of this pit, a pot should be kept. Over this pot another earthen pot should be kept with face upwards. There should be a hole at the bottom of the upper earthen pot to allow the neck of a bottle to come out. The bottle, which is wrapped with seven layers of mud-smeared cloth, should be filled up with medicine and its mouth should be covered with the help of an iron net of very fine mesh. The remaining space over the upper vessel should be filled up with charcoal and ignited. Because of this heat, the oil of the ingredients inside the bottle will start exudating and gradually through the iron net this oil will trickle down to the vessel kept at the bottom of the pit. It can be used even for preparing oil from some oil seeds like *bhallātaka* (*Semecarpus anacardium* Linn. f.). This is called *Pātāla yantra.*

PĀTĀLA YANTRA
(APPARATUS FOR UNDER GROUND EXTRACTION)

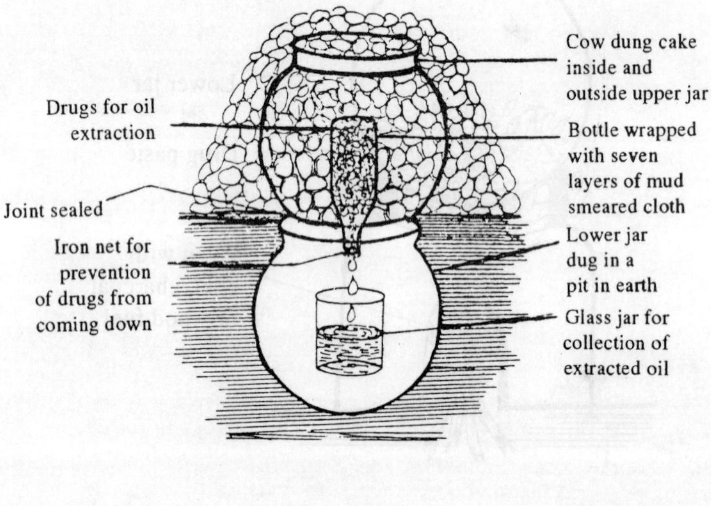

FIGURE - 20

Khalva Yantra or Pestle and Mortar

Pestle and mortar are very commonly used in processing mercury and other metals. They are of different shapes and sizes. The mortar can be round or oblong. It can be shallow or deep. This is made of black stone in general but for specific purposes, mortar and pestle prepared of iron, agate, etc., are also used. The size and shape of the pestle also vary. This is called *Khalva yantra.*

At times, the mortar during the preparation of the medicine has to be kept over fire. Since stone mortar will not be able to stand the effect of the heat and is likely to crack, usually for this purpose, iron mortar and pestle are used. This is called *Tapta khalva yantra.*

TAPTA KHALVA YANTRA
(HOT MORTAR AND PESTLE)

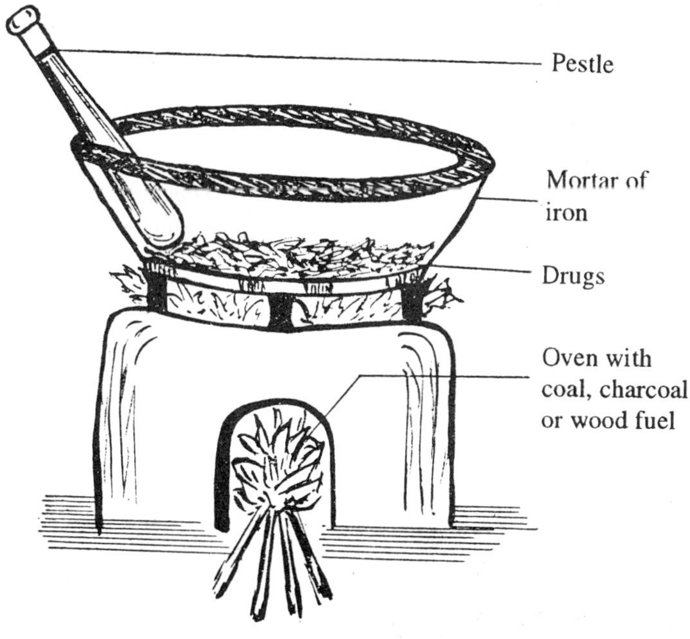

FIGURE - 21

In *Rasa śāstra* several other equipments are used. Equipments described above are only the commonly used ones.

Śarāva Sampuṭa (Enclosure with Two Earthen Plates)

If any metal, like gold, is to be reduced to *bhasma* form, then first of all it is triturated with other prescribed drugs and made to a paste. From out of this paste, small round and flat cakes *(cakrikās)* of about one inch in diameter are prepared. These cakes are then dried in the sun. Thereafter, these cakes are kept inside two earthen plates and the joint of these plates is sealed by wrapping seven layers of mud-smeared cloth. Then this is dried in the sun before cooking in a *puṭa*. This is called *Śarāva sampuṭa.*

ŚARĀVA SAMPUṬA
ENCLOSURE WITH TWO EARTHEN PLATES

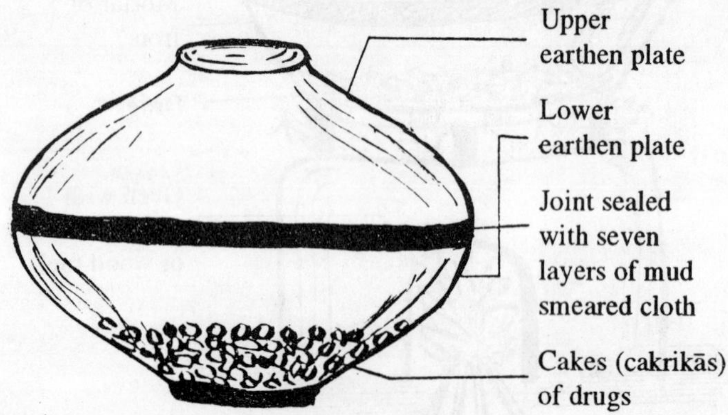

FIGURE - 22

BIBLIOGRAPHY

Ācārya, Yādavajī Trikamjī. *Rasāmṛtam* (Banārasa : Motīlāla Banārasīdāsa, 1951).

Ārya, Satyendrakumar. *Āyurvedīya Rasaśāstra Kā Udbhava evaṃ Vikāsa*. Ist ed. (Varanasi : Krishnadas Academy, 1984).

Bhaṭṭa, Śrīkṛṣṇarāma. *Siddha-bheṣaja-maṇimālā* (Jayapura: Īśānacandra Bhaṭṭa, 1968).

Caube, Dattarāma. *Bṛhad Rasarāja Sundara*. 2nd ed. (Vārānasi: Caukhambhā Oriyanṭaliya, 1985).

Chopra, R. N. et. al. *Glossary of Indian Medicinal Plants* (New Delhi: Council of Scientific & Industrial Research, 1956).

Dash, Bhagwan. *Fundamentals of Ayurvedic Medicine*. 4th ed. (Delhi: Bansal & Co., 1984).

Dash, Bhagwan; Kashyap, Lalitesh. *Materia Medica of Ayurveda based on Ayurveda Saukhyam* of Ṭoḍarānanda. (New Delhi : Concept Publishing Company, 1980).

Dvivedī, Vāsudeva Mūlaśaṅkara. *Pāradavijñānīyam* (Datiyā: Śarmā Āyurveda Mandira, 1969).

Govinda Bhagavatpāda. *Rasa-hṛdaya-tantra* (Kaleḍā-Kṛshṇagopāla: Kṛṣhṇa-Gopāla Āyurveda Bhavana, 1958).

Gupta, Nirañjana Prasāda. *Pārada Saṃhitā*. (Bambai: Khemarāja Śrīkṛṣhṇadāsa, 1926).

Kutumbiah, P. *Ancient Indian Medicine*. (Bombay: Orient Longmans, 1962).

Mahdihassan, S. *Indian Alchemy or Rasāyana* (New Delhi: Institute of History of Medicine and Medical Research, 1977).

Mookerjee, Bhudeb. *Rasa-jala-nidhi*. Vol. I-V. 2nd ed. (Varanasi: Srigokul Mudranalaya, 1984).

Mukhopadhyaya, Girindranath. *History of Indian Medicine* (New Delhi: Oriental Books Reprint Corporation, 1974).

Nityanātha Siddha. *Rasāyana Khaṇḍa of Rasaratnākara*. 2nd ed. (Varanasi: Chaukambha Amarabharati Prakashan, 1982).

Oak, P. N. *World Vedic Heritage*. 1st ed. (New Delhi: P. N. Oak, 1984).

Pāṇḍeya, Badarī Nārāyaṇ. *Āyurvedīya Rasaśāstra.* Ist ed. (Lakhanau: Avadha Prakāśana, 1978).

Panta Tārādatta (ed.). *Rasārṇavam or Rasatantram* (Benares : The Chowkhamba Sanskrit Series Office, 1939).

Radhakrishna Shastri, S.V. (ed.). *Anandakandam* (Tanjore: T.M S.S.M. Library, 1952).

Ray, Prafulla Chandra. *History of Chemistry in Ancient and Medieval India* (Calcutta : Indian Chemical Society, 1956).

Śarmā, Sadānanda. *Rasataraṅgiṇī.* 5th ed. (Banārasa : Motīlāla Banārasīdāsa, 1953).

Śarmā, Hariprapanna. *Rasayogasāgara.* Vol. I-II. 2nd ed. (Varanasi: Krishnadas Academy, 1983).

Śarmā, Hari Śaṅkara. *Śulva Śāstram* (Jāmanagara: Āyurvedīya Snātakottara Śikṣaṇa Kendram, 1961).

Seal, Brajendranath. *The Positive Sciences of Ancient Hindus* (Delhi : Motilal Banarasi Dass, 1958).

Shanmuga Velan, A. *Siddhar's Science of Longevity and Kalpa Medicine of India* (Madras : Śakthi Nilayam, 1963).

Sharma, P.V. *Āyurveda Kā Vaijñānika Itihāsa.* Ist ed. (Varanasi : Chowkhamba Orientalia, 1975).

Sharma, P.V. *Dravya-guṇa Vijñana.* 3rd ed. (Varanasi : Chaukhambha Sanskrit Sansthan, 1975).

Sharma, R.K.; Dash, Bhagwan. *Caraka Saṃhitā: text with English Translation and Critical exposition based on Cakrapāṇi Datta's Āyurveda Dīpikā.* Vols. I-II. (Varanasi) : Chowkhambha Sanskrit Series Office, 1976).

Sherwood Taylor, F. *The Alchemists, Founders of Modern Chemistry* (Melbourne: William Heinemann Ltd., 1958).

Singh, Thakur Balwant; Chunekar, K.C. *Glossary of Vegetable Drugs in Bṛhattrayī.* Ist ed. (Varanasi : Chowkhambha Sanskrit Series Office, 1972).

Somadeva, *Rasendra Cūḍāmaṇi.* (Varanasi: Chawkhambhā Oriyanṭaliā, 1984).

Triveda, D.S. *Indian Chronology.* (Bombay: Bharatiya Vidya Bhavan, 1963).

Upādhyāya, Mādhava. *Āyurvedaprakāśa* (Nāgapura: Śrīdhanvantaryyāurveda-mahāvidyālaya, 1943).

Vāgbhaṭacārya. *Rasaratna Samuccaya* (Varanasi: Chowkhambha Sanskrit Series Office, 1961).

Yaśodhara. *Rasaprakāśa Sudhākara* (Varanasi : Chaukhambha Oriyanṭaliā, 1983).

INDEX

INDEX